LANGUAGES AND LINGUISTICS

THE EFFECTS OF DRUGS ON VERBAL FLUENCY

LANGUAGES AND LINGUISTICS

Additional books in this series can be found on Nova's website under the Series tab.

Additional E-books in this series can be found on Nova's website under the E-books tab.

THE EFFECTS OF DRUGS
ON VERBAL FLUENCY

DARIO ZANETTI

MARIA R. PIRAS

MARINELLA D'ONOFRIO

CATERINA F. BAGELLA

PAOLA LAI

LAURA FANCELLU

SUSANNA M. NUVOLI

AND GIANPIETRO SECHI

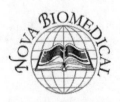

Nova Science Publishers, Inc.
New York

MW

For permission to use material from this book please contact us:
Telephone 631-231-7269; Fax 631-231-8175
Web Site: http://www.novapublishers.com

NOTICE TO THE READER

The Publisher has taken reasonable care in the preparation of this book, but makes no expressed or implied warranty of any kind and assumes no responsibility for any errors or omissions. No liability is assumed for incidental or consequential damages in connection with or arising out of information contained in this book. The Publisher shall not be liable for any special, consequential, or exemplary damages resulting, in whole or in part, from the readers' use of, or reliance upon, this material.

Independent verification should be sought for any data, advice or recommendations contained in this book. In addition, no responsibility is assumed by the publisher for any injury and/or damage to persons or property arising from any methods, products, instructions, ideas or otherwise contained in this publication.

This publication is designed to provide accurate and authoritative information with regard to the subject matter covered herein. It is sold with the clear understanding that the Publisher is not engaged in rendering legal or any other professional services. If legal or any other expert assistance is required, the services of a competent person should be sought. FROM A DECLARATION OF PARTICIPANTS JOINTLY ADOPTED BY A COMMITTEE OF THE AMERICAN BAR ASSOCIATION AND A COMMITTEE OF PUBLISHERS.

LIBRARY OF CONGRESS CATALOGING-IN-PUBLICATION DATA

Available upon Request
ISBN: 978-1-61668-759-5

Published by Nova Science Publishers, Inc. ✛ New York

6/13/11

CONTENTS

PREFACE

In this book, in the light of the recent discoveries in the field of cognitive neuroscience, functional neuroanatomy, and neurochemistry, we discuss the neuroanatomical and the neurochemical bases of speech and language. Afterwards, we reviewed the relevant literature concerning the influence of drugs and other related substances on speech and language, with emphasis on verbal fluency, as well as the mechanisms of drug-related fluency and the pharmacotherapy of aphasia. Furthermore, we discuss the effects of topiramate in a patient with a post-traumatic, light form of non-fluent dysphasia.

Chapter 1

INTRODUCTION

The idea of using drugs to improve speech and language disorders in neurologic patients is not new indeed, in the 1950s, Luria suggested to use anticholinesterase drugs in stroke patients with aphasia [de Boissezon et al., 2007]. Nevertheless, the neurochemistry of speech and language and the pharmacology of aphasia and other speech and language disorders remains a domain of neuroscience still in its early infancy. The neuroanatomical loops involved in the control of verbal fluency have recently been studied in humans through functional neuroimaging. These include many cortical and subcortical polysynaptic pathways mainly in the left hemisphere, with different neurotransmitters, such as serotonin, dopamine, noradrenaline, acetylcholine and GABA, proposed for the pathways regulating verbal fluency. In consequence, a myriad of drugs commonly used in clinical practice, also with very different pharmacological action, may affect the complex neuroanatomical/ biochemical network regulating speech and language and thus influence verbal fluency and other linguistic abilities, such as syntax and semantics, either in a positive or a negative way. The implicated drugs include the old and new antiepileptic agents, neuroleptics, dopaminergic drugs, β-blockers, antidepressants, benzodiazepines and stimulant agents, such as cocaine and methylphenidate.

Chapter 2

NEUROANATOMY OF SPEECH AND LANGUAGE

At the end of the 19th century, clinical studies on epileptic patients by Jackson, and on aphasic patients by Freud, Dax, Lichtheim, Broca, and Wernicke showed that various linguistic functions were controlled by specific cortical areas. In particular, they found out that the major cortical structures involved in language are the inferior left frontal gyrus (Broca's area or Brodmann's areas 44 and 45), which is responsible for articulated speech, the left posterior, superior, middle temporal cortex and the inferior parietal cortex (Wernicke's area or Brodmann's areas 22, 37, 39, and 40), which are responsible for understanding spoken language and the arcuate fasciculus, which connects Wernicke's area and Broca's area. Moreover, they found out that there is a functional asymmetry for language in the two hemispheres [Wernicke, 1874; Caplan, 1998; Kandel et al., 2000; Cacciari, 2001; Ladavas & Berti, 2002; Catani et al., 2005].

But, since the first cases of aphasia described by the French physician Paul Broca in 1861 and by the German neurologist Carl Wernicke in 1874, science has made great strides. Today, scientists use those models which view both language and brain in hierarchical terms. In fact, behaviour is considered to be the result of the functioning of successive levels of the nervous system and not, as traditionally believed the result of complex behaviors which took their origin from simple components. In addition, it is believed that language which is a particular form of behavior is the result of the cooperation between the nervous system and the psyche [Caplan, 1998; Cacciari, 2001; Ladavas & Berti, 2002].

In the last few decades, the attention of most scientists has moved from the idea of finding the exact anatomical localization of language in the brain, in the attempt to understand the relationship between language and the different functions of the nervous system. Instead of regarding Broca's and Wernicke's area as the main cortical language areas, they can be seen as areas which are intensively used for speech and language [Cacciari, 2001].

According to the most common neuroscientific and neuropsychological models, in all right-handed individuals verbal abilities and the ability to do fine movements are concentrated in the left cerebral hemisphere. As the left hemisphere is the part of the brain in which symbolic and analytical processes are elaborated, it is also responsible for the elaboration of language. Though the left hemisphere contains prevalently those areas which are involved in speech and language, it seems that it plays an important role not only in the elaboration of speech and language, but also in the elaboration of all those cognitive functions which are implicitly mediated by language. In the past, it was believed that the right hemisphere did not play an important function in the elaboration of language, as according to many neuroscientists, it was not implicated in the elaboration of symbolic representations. But nowadays, it seems that the right hemisphere is even more important in the elaboration of spatial and perceptive tasks than the left hemisphere [Cacciari, 2001]. As shown in Table 1, there are abilities which are bound to one cortical hemisphere rather than to the other hemisphere [Cacciari, 2001]. But, in fact, even the right hemisphere plays a rather important role in the elaboration of those processes which are bound to speech and language, and it accomplishes various important tasks which are related to particular linguistic aspects both during childhood and adulthood. In particular, the right hemisphere is important for communicative and emotional prosody, such as stress of words, timing and intonation, and for figurative aspects of language. In addition, this hemisphere plays a role in the pragmatics and semantics of language, but above all in the organization of narrative aspects and symbolic representations of language, but not in that of single words [Cacciari, 2001].

The manifold of results which have been accumulated in the last thirty years of neuroscientific research suggest that the right hemisphere participates actively in the elaboration of language, and moreover they suggest that the elaboration of language happens in a more distributed way in the two hemispheres. So, according to this model, the two hemispheres work together, and they elaborate the entire incoming linguistic information [Cacciari, 2001].

Further studies proved that the cortical regions involved in the processing of speech and language go far beyond the two classical language areas of

Broca and Wernicke. In fact, almost the entire neocortex of the left hemisphere is involved in these processes, including the temporal, parietal, prefrontal, and frontal lobes (figure 1) [for a detailed overview see: Démonet et al., 2005; Vigneau et al., 2006].

Table 1. Cognitive abilities, which are more lateralized in the two cerebral hemispheres

Left-hemisphere dominance	General functions	Right-hemisphere dominance
Words	VISION	Geometric patterns
Letters		Faces
		Emotional expression
Language sounds	AUDITION	Nonlanguage sounds
		Music
	TOUCH	Tactual patterns
		Braille
Complex movement	MOVEMENT	Movement in spatial patterns
Verbal memory	MEMORY	Nonverbal memory
Speech	LANGUAGE	Emotional content
Reading		
Writing		
Arithmetic		
	SPATIAL ABILITY	Geometry
		Direction
		Distance
		Mental rotation of shapes

Therefore, this wide distribution suggests that language is not only localized in Broca's and Wernicke's area, even if clinical reports sometimes seem to prove the contrary. For instance, the analysis of brain imaging data of text comprehension through recently developed meta-analysis methods let to the identification of a network of fronto-temporal brain regions extending far beyond the perisylvian language cortex [Ferstl et al., 2008]. This newly developed analysis method showed that in addition to the contribution of the left inferior frontal and posterior superior temporal regions, there is also activation in the anterior temporal lobes [Ferstl et al., 2008]. Complex cognitive activities such as speech and language are the result of a continuous interaction between a large number of different cortical regions localized in the two cerebral hemispheres which are connected through neuronal pathways. The elaboration of language is based on a hierarchical organization.

Furthermore, the classical language areas are not unitary modules, but on the contrary, they are complex areas arranged in clusters, and each cluster is formed by different functional components [Cacciari, 2001].

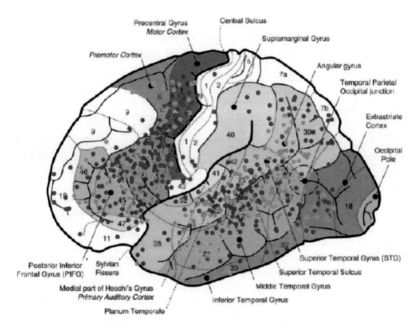

Figure 1. The main brain regions involved in language processing are colored in grey. Numbers indicate Brodmann's areas separated by dotted lines. The colour dots indicate the activation peak for phonology (blue), semantics (red) and syntactic (green) processing [Figure used with permission and adapted from Démonet et al., 2005; Vigneau et al., 2006].

Today, most neuroscientists believe that cognitive functions such as speech and language are distributed among different cortical regions in both hemispheres, and it has been realized that their neuronal organization is far more complex than believed. Without doubt, the classical model derived from the work of Broca, Wernicke, Lichtheim, and Geschwind has been very useful as a heuristic model which has stimulated numerous studies and as a clinical model useful in practice for clinical diagnosis. Nevertheless, according to most modern neuroscientists, undoubtedly the classical model is empirical wrong. In fact, it cannot justify the range of aphasic syndromes, and its linguistic foundations are impoverished and conceptually underspecified. Furthermore, the classical model is anatomically underspecified, i.e. its anatomical affirmations are not true anymore. It has become clear, that Broca's aphasia is not caused by a mere damage to Broca's area, Wernicke's aphasia is not caused by simple damage to Wernicke's area and conduction aphasia is not caused by only damage to the arcuate fasciculus. Moreover, conduction aphasia is no longer classified as a disconnection syndrome. And, it is scientifically proved, that the classical speech-related regions are not homogeneous from an anatomical or functional point of view [Cacciari, 2001; Poeppel & Hickok, 2004].

A recent diffusion tensor magnetic resonance imaging study [Catani et al., 2005] has revealed the existence of two parallel pathways connecting the temporal and frontal regions of the left hemisphere: 1) a direct pathway (arcuate fasciculus; long segment) anticipated by Wernicke and 2) a newly discovered indirect pathway connecting temporal with parietal (posterior segment), and parietal with frontal regions (anterior segment). The data obtained by this brain imaging study suggests that the connection between frontal and temporal language regions is far more complex than previously thought, and furthermore it revealed the existence of a perisylvian language network. These neuroanatomical findings are supported by clinical evidence, too. According to Catani et al. [2005], it seems that the indirect pathway is associated to semantically-based language functions, such as auditory comprehension and vocalization of semantic content, whereas the direct pathway is associated to phonologically based language functions, such as automatic repetition. This does not mean that these functions are only restricted to perisylvian areas, but that, within the parallel pathways, they are automatically dissociable. Moreover, it seems that the distribution of the arcuate fibre terminations extends far beyond Broca's area (Brodmann's area 44 and 45), and that it includes part of the middle frontal gyrus and inferior precentral gyrus. This demonstrates that Broca's area is surrounded by cortical regions which are specialized in higher language (or linguistic) functions. Catani et al. [2005] call this extended region "Broca's territory". In addition, the same can be said for Wernicke's area, too. This study suggests that the posterior temporal and inferior parietal region of Wernicke's area is densely connected, but they have to be seen as two distinct anatomical areas. Furthermore, it seems that the distribution of the fibre terminations in the posterior region is wider than previously thought, including the posterior part of both the superior and middle temporal gyrus. Catani et al. [2005] call this extended region "Wernicke's territory". This study not only emphasizes the importance of the inferior parietal cortex as a separate language area, but it also shows that the inferior parietal cortex is densely connected to Broca's and Wernicke's area through the indirect pathway.

The cortico-centric view of language is supplemented by models that additionally propose language-related functions for subcortical structures, such as the thalamus and the basal ganglia. These theoretical models are not only supported by various clinical studies of patients with an atypical aphasia due to cerebrovascular damage to the basal ganglia [Brunner et al., 1982; Damasio et al., 1982; Naesser et al., 1982; Wallesch et al., 1983; Cappa, 1997; Nadeau & Crosson, 1997] and by patients with language impairments caused by neurodegenerative diseases involving the basal ganglia, such as Parkinson's disease [Cummings et al., 1988; Illes et al., 1989; Copland, 2001, 2003] and Huntington's disease [Gordon and Illes, 1987], but also by various and recent neurofunctional studies which investigated the role of the basal ganglia and that of the thalamus in the elaboration and processing of language [Ketteler et al., 2008; Christensen et al, 2008]. But nevertheless, the exact role of the thalamus and of the basal ganglia in the elaboration and processing of language still remains unclear, and there is an ongoing debate whether these subcortical structures are involved in language processing or not. For instance, according to Crosson [1997, 2002], the basal ganglia and in particular the thalamus seem to play only a slight role in the elaboration and processing of language. On the contrary, Wallesch [1997] suggested that cortico-striato-pallido-thalamo-cortical loops are not only involved in motor pathways, but they are also involved in cognitive language functions. According to Alexander [1994], and Bhatia and Marsden [1994], there are two main neuronal pathways of the basal ganglia which play a rather important role in the regulation of movement and language, namely the cortico-striato-pallido-thalamo-cortical loop and the cortico-striato-subthalamo-thalamo-cortical loop. The first loop, also known as the direct pathway, collects and elaborates the information coming from all cortical lobes. This pathway has an excitatory influence on the frontal lobe (positive feedback). Whereas, the second loop also known as the indirect loop or outer putamen-pallidus-pathway has an inhibitory function, since it inhibits the frontal lobe (negative feedback) by suppressing all those motor and psyche schemes which are in direct competition with movement or cognitive action. In particular, it seems that the basal ganglia may play a rather important role in what might be called the executive semantic functions, i.e. they are part of a neural system which monitors the cortical parallel processing and which selects semantically-adequate lexical units [Wallesch & Papagno, 1988]. Moreover, it seems that the basal ganglia are implicated in syntactic processing, too, and in this case they are part of fronto-striatal circuitry which not only provide the executive resources needed to understand complex syntax [Grossman, 1999], but also process syntactic rules [Lieberman et al., 1990; Natsopoulos et al., 1991, 1993; McNamara et al., 1996]. The analog to memory concept, which is summarized in the "declarative/procedural model" [Ullman et al., 1997; Ullman, 2001; Pinker & Ullman, 2002] proposes that the basal ganglia are part of a neural system which controls rule-governed grammatical operations. This model makes a clear and sharp distinction between procedural and declarative memory system. The implicit memory or fronto-striatal procedural memory system is involved in grammatical rule use, while the explicit memory or temporo-parietal declarative memory system is involved in explicit memory of arbitrary facts. The basal ganglia in combination with the thalamus trigger the cortex for language production; it seems that the thalamus is needed for particular linguistic sub-processes, for instance semantic search mechanism and making semantic choices from among multiple lexical possibilities [Ketteler et al., 2008]. It was seen that subcortical-electrical stimulation during neurosurgery [Fabbro, 1999] sometimes induces the patients to speak involuntarily. This suggests that only specific structures of the basal ganglia and of the thalamus are implicated in verbal expression, and moreover it suggests that the cortex has the function to regulate the final phases of the language production process as soon as verbal expression is activated. These neurophysiological experiments have revealed that the subcortical structures which are actively involved in word and sentence production are the head of the nucleus caudatus and most of the anterior nuclei of the thalamus. As a matter of fact, electrical stimulation of the head of the nucleus caudatus leads patients, who are awake during neurosurgery, to produce sentences which have nothing to do with the experimental or clinical procedure. In addition, electrical stimulation of the most anterior left thalamic nuclei leads the subjects to a strong desire to speak, but the uttered words or sentences are totally out of the given context. Important to mention is that there is a high concentration of noradrenaline in the left thalamus. From a biochemical point of view, this neurotransmitter has a biological action very similar to that of caffeine and cocaine which increase the desire to speak and make the conversation more fluent and lucid. Various clinical studies have revealed that lesions in the basal ganglia of the left hemisphere may cause the following language disorders:

1. non-fluent aphasia with a general reduction in spontaneous speech;
2. voice disorders, such as "foreign accent syndrome";
3. presence of semantic and verbal paraphasias, which normally are found only in fluent aphasia;

4. signs of echolalia and perseverations;
5. in general, repetition and comprehension are not affected;
6. writing disorders.

Whereas, lesions to the thalamus of the left hemisphere may cause the following language disorders:

1. verbal expression is altered, speech is fluent and the patient is affected by a severe anomia, while comprehension is in general less compromised;
2. verbal, semantic paraphasias and neologisms;
3. mild comprehension deficit, whereas repetition is spared;
4. disorders in reading, writing, arithmetic, and long-term verbal memory.

In 1917, the neurologist Gordon Holmes described a new form of language disorder caused by cerebellar lesions; these patients had significant speech motor deficits. He called this new form of language disorder ataxic dysarthria. Indeed, damage to the cerebellum may affect the motor production of speech, and therefore patients affected by cerebellar disorder frequently speak in a slow way and make many and severe errors in phonation and articulation. Furthermore, the voice of such patients sounds irregular due to the tremor of the organs involved in speech articulation. It seems that the cerebellum has two major functions within the verbal domain [Ackermann, 2008]: 1) it subserves the online sequencing of syllables into fast, smooth and rhythmically organized larger utterances, and 2) it is involved in the temporal organization of internal speech. According to Ackermann [2008], internal speech can be seen as a sort of prearticulatory verbal code; and its impairment could somehow explain some of those perceptual and cognitive disorders seen in patients with cerebellar damage. Neuroanatomical and neurophysiological investigations [Fabbro, 1999] have shown that the left cerebral cortex is directly connected with the right cerebellar hemisphere through a neuronal pathway. Recent neurofunctional and lesion studies [Fabbro, 1999] have shown an activation of the lateral cerebellar hemispheres during language processing, while the vermis and the paraverminal regions are implicated in motor aspects of speech. Various positron emission tomography (PET) studies [Fabbro, 1999] which investigated the activation of neuronal structures during the performance of cognitive tasks have shown that there is an activation of the right cerebellar hemisphere during the execution of purely linguistic tasks.

Finally, other neurofunctional studies [Fabbro, 1999] have revealed that the cerebellum participates in speech perception as well. In addition, it seems that some structures of the cerebellum, in particular the neocerebellum, may play an important part in the regulation of nonmotor cognitive functions.

Chapter 3

NEUROCHEMICAL BASES OF
SPEECH AND LANGUAGE

Today, it is known that the brain is formed by neurofunctional units which are the neural cells or neurons, and by supporting cells which are the glia. Moreover, these neural cells tend to form neuronal groups, and some of these neuronal groups are connected together and form neuronal circuits[1], while a system is formed by a neuronal circuit and has well-defined functions, such as hearing or seeing. Every neural cell elaborates and transmits information, i.e. it receives information from other neurons, elaborates the obtained information and afterwards transmits it to thousands of other neurons. Without any doubt, the most important characteristic of neurons is that of sending information by means of electrical signals through extension of single cells (axons). The dendrites connect the cell body of a neuron to other neural cells through the synapses, whereas the main function of the axon is that of sending information to other structures. In the vicinity of the synapses between the neural cells, electrical impulses release neurotransmitters which are stored in the presynaptic axonal terminal. These neurotransmitters modify the electrical activity of a postsynaptic neuron [Cooper et al., 2003; Siegel et al., 2006].

---

[1] Neuronal circuits are formed by excitatory and inhibitory mechanisms whose complexity depends on the type of function they subserve.

THE PRIMARY NEUROTRANSMITTERS

Glutamate, γ-Aminobutyric Acid and Glycine

There are two general categories of amino acid neurotransmitters. These neurotransmitters are classified on the basis of their functional actions, i.e. on the one hand, there are excitatory amino acid neurotransmitters (glutamate [Glu], aspartate [Asp], cysteate and homocysteate), which depolarize neurons in the mammalian central nervous system (CNS), and on the other hand, there are inhibitory amino acid neurotransmitters (γ-aminobutyric acid [GABA], glycine [Gly], taurine and β-alanine), which hyperpolarize neurons in the mammalian CNS [Cooper et al., 2003; Siegel et al., 2006].

The amino acid glutamate not only mediates almost every fast excitatory neurotransmission in the CNS, but also excites nearly every neural cell of it and is the main mediator of sensory information, motor coordination, emotions, and cognition, such as language, memory formation, and memory retrieval. Glutamate is used as a neurotransmitter by almost 90% of the neural cells of the brain, and about 80-90% of the synapses are glutamatergic. There is a high concentration of glutamate in brain gray matter structures which varies between 10 and 15 µmol/g of tissue, while the concentration of glutamate in white matter structures is a bit lower (4-10 µmol/g of tissue). Glutamate is involved in many reactions in the CNS. This neurotransmitter is not only a precursor for GABA in GABAergic neurons and for glutamine in glial cells, but also a component of proteins and peptides, such as glutathione (γ-glutamyl-cysteinyl-glycine). So, it can be said that glutamate is not only found in the cytosol and mitochondria of almost every cell of the CNS (neuronal and glial), but also in the cell body and its processes. Glutamate is stored in synaptic vesicles as transmitter glutamate in glutamatergic neurons. Learning is one of the most important characteristics of our behavior. This process must have an anatomical substrate; that is, our brain must be modified somehow in order to allow the storage of the information/knowledge which is to be learnt. It is believed that these particular changes which allow the storage of information take place at the synaptic level by means of particular biochemical and electrophysiological processes called "synaptic plasticity". But it is not known whether these changes take place on the presynaptic or on the postsynaptic side of the synaptic cleft. From an electrophysiological point of view, there are two phenomena which may be involved in the learning mechanism at the synaptic level, i.e. the long-term potentiation (LTP) and the long-term depression (LTD) of synaptic efficacy. In general, glutamatergic synapses are axo-dendritic synapses or axo-axonal synapses, but glutamate receptors can also be found in astrocytes, oligodendrocytes and in microglia. There are two main glutamate receptors, i.e. ionotropic receptors (ionotropic receptors are cation channels themselves) and metabotropic receptors (metabotropic receptors influence indirectly the activity of ion channels). The ionotropic receptors are N-methyl-D-aspartate (NMDA), α-amino-3-hydroxy-5-methyl-4-isoxazole propionic acid (AMPA) and kainate (KA). There are eight metabotropic glutamate receptors (mGluR1-mGluR8), and their main function is to modulate synaptic transmission [Cooper et al., 2003; Siegel et al., 2006].

The inhibitory neurotransmitter GABA is found in high concentrations in many brain regions and in the spinal cord, but is absent or present only in trace amounts in peripheral nerve tissue. GABA is stored in vesicles in the presynaptic terminals and released into the synaptic cleft. There are two distinct classes of GABA receptors, i.e. GABA$_A$ receptors (ionotropic) and GABA$_B$ receptors (metabotropic). These receptors vary in their pharmacological, electrophysiological, and biochemical properties. GABA$_A$ receptors are the main inhibitory neurotransmitter receptors of the CNS and the site of action of many clinically significant drugs. GABA$_B$ receptors are mediator of both postsynaptic and presynaptic inhibition, and they are coupled to G proteins. The structure of GABA$_B$ receptors is very similar to the one of the metabotropic glutamate receptors [Cooper et al., 2003; Siegel et al., 2006].

Another important inhibitory neurotransmitter is glycine (simplest amino acid) which is primarily found in the spinal cord and brainstem, but glycinergic interneurons can also be found in the retina, the auditory system and in those brain areas which are implicated in the processing and elaboration of sensory information. Glycine and GABA mediate almost every fast inhibitory neurotransmission in the CNS by inhibiting neuronal firing through Cl$^-$ channels [Cooper et al., 2003; Siegel et al., 2006].

Neuromodulators and Hormones

In general, the different neurotransmitters do not work alone; in fact, their activity is regulated by various chemical substances, i.e. by neuromodulators.

There are two main classes of neuromodulators:

1. peptides (β-endorphin, enkephalins, neurotensin etc.);
2. hormones.

Neuromodulators can be either excitatory or inhibitory agents, and in general, they produce changes in conductance or membrane potential [Cooper et al., 2003; Siegel et al., 2006].

Besides the amino acid neurotransmitters, there are also catecholaminergic, cholinergic, and serotonergic neurotransmitters with their equivalent systems [Cooper et al., 2003; Siegel et al., 2006].

Catecholamines

The catecholamines which are 1) dopamine (DA), 2) norepinephrine (NE) and 3) epinephrine (E) are neurotransmitters and/or hormones in the periphery and in the CNS. In fact, NE is not only found in the CNS, but also in postganglionic, sympathetic neurons. DA, which is the precursor of NE, is active in the periphery and acts as a neurotransmitter in numerous important pathways in the CNS. E is a hormone which is released from the adrenal gland, but small quantities of this hormone can be found in the CNS, as well, above all in the brainstem. Its main function is that of stimulating the various catecholamine receptors in different organs. Catecholamines are stored in storage vesicles which have a high density within nerve terminals, but low concentrations of catecholamines are also found in the cytosol [Cooper et al., 2003; Siegel et al., 2006].

Dopamine is synthesized in the pigmented neurons of the substantia nigra (SN) and the ventral tegmental area (VTA). The dopaminergic system is formed by three main ascending systems, i.e. by the striatonigral tract (the fibres which have their origin in the SN project to the corpus striatum [caudate and putamen]), the mesolimbic system (in this case, the fibres ascend from the SN and medial VTA to limbic sites and to the cingulated gyrus) and the mesocortical system (the fibres which have their origin in the anteromedial tegmentum and VTA not only project to the striatum, but also to the amygdala, basal forebrain and medial frontal lobes, including the supplementary motor area[2] [SMA] and the prefrontal cortex). The density of forebrain dopamine innervation diminishes in a rostrocaudal gradient, and for that reason, only trace amounts of DA are present in the occipital brain regions. The brain regions with the highest density of dopamine innervation are the primary

---

[2] Clinical studies reported that lesions to the supplementary motor area cause alteration of verbal fluency and impairment in the initiation of output. The aphasic syndrome caused by such lesions is classified as a transcortical motor aphasia [Klein et al., 2004].

motor cortex, the SMA, and the prefrontal and inferior parietal areas. Moreover, it seems that dopaminergic activity is greater in the left hemisphere than in the right one, particularly in the left forebrain. So, it can be said that DA fibres innervate prefrontal, motor and association areas in the cortex. These pathways control the initiation and maintenance of complex motor activity, attentional switching, and the production of sequential voluntary motor activity. In addition, in the human brain DA interacts with five different receptors, which are the so called D1-like (D1 and D5) and D2-like (D2, D3 and D4) receptors [Cooper et al., 2003; Klein et al., 2004; McNamara et al., 2004; Siegel et al., 2006].

In general, this catecholaminergic neurotransmitter is associated with the neurodegenerative disorder Parkinson's disease (PD); in this case, there is a progressive loss of the dopamine producing neurons of the SN. It has been reported that Parkinson's patients have characteristic speech and language abnormalities. This seems to confirm the hypothesis that DA is involved in language functions [Cooper et al., 2003; Klein et al., 2004; McNamara et al., 2004; Siegel et al., 2006].

In 2000, McNamara and Durso published a review concerning speech and language disorders in non-demented Parkinson's patients. They found out that besides deficits in fluency, in syntactic comprehension and in prefrontal control of attention, Parkinson's patients have also motor speech disorders. Furthermore, according to McNamara and Durso, speech and language disorders which are similar to those observed in patients with Broca's aphasia can also be found in Parkinson's patients, if there is a disruption of DA pathways between the basal ganglia and the prefrontal cortex.

In summary, it can be said that DA is involved in various fundamental speech and language functions, such as initiation, fluency, naming (in particular lexical retrieval) and language content. Furthermore, it seems that dopamine influences emotional, pragmatic and prosodic functions, too. These speech and language functions are elaborated in the right prefrontal brain regions [Klein et al., 2004; McNamara et al., 2004].

Norepinephrine which is synthesized in the locus coeruleus (LC) in the pontine brainstem is stored in synaptic vesicles in nerve endings and released through exocytosis. Noradrenergic neurons give off many collaterals which innervate various cortical brain regions; in fact, they innervate every major region of the forebrain as well as the primary sensory and motor cortex. The density of forebrain NE innervation diminishes in a rostrocaudal gradient, and therefore only small traces of NE are found in the posterior brain regions. As a matter of fact, the brain regions with a dense noradrenergic innervation are the primary somatosensory and the motor regions, which are densely innervated in all six layers, whereas temporal and primary visual cortices have a lower innervation density. It is known that damage to the dorsolateral prefrontal cortex not only uninhibits the firing of locus ceruleus neurons but also impairs the regulation of the LC. In fact, the prefrontal cortex seems to be the only cortical structure which supplies cortical afferents to the LC. Therefore, it can be pointed out that both the prefrontal cortex and the ascending noradrenergic system influence the processing properties of each other, for instance if there is an impairment in the functioning of the prefrontal cortex, there will be an impairment in the functioning of the ascending noradrenergic system, as well, and vice versa. It has been observed that after a stroke, there is a fall of NE levels in the cerebrum, brainstem, cerebellum, and cerebrospinal fluid which is most clear ipsilateral to the side of the lesion. Moreover, it is known that NE is involved in the regulation of prefrontal functions and of attentional switching. This suggests that NE could also influence perseverative responding in the verbal sphere [Cooper et al., 2003; Klein et al., 2004; McNamara et al., 2004; Siegel et al., 2006].

Acetylcholine

Acetylcholine (ACh) has a broad distribution in the nervous system. ACh not only favours every motor transmission in vertebrates, but is also the most important transmitter for peripheral ganglia and mediator of parasympathetic actions of the autonomic nervous system. Furthermore, ACh is a leading neurotransmitter in the CNS. As a matter of fact, the principal forebrain source of cholinergic innervation includes various nuclei of the basal forebrain, which are the nucleus basalis of Meynert (nbM), the horizontal and vertical diagonal bands of Broca, the substantia innominata and the medial septal nucleus. These nuclei form the basal forebrain cholinergic system, and they (in particular the nbM) are associated with Alzheimer's disease (AD). In addition, there is a second group of cholinergic neurons which is localized in the brainstem near the peduncolopontine tegmental nucleus and the laterodorsal pontine tegmentum. Even if the majority of basal forebrain cholinergic neurons send diffusely their afferents all over the cortex, these neurons get inputs from only a small number of areas, which comprises the reticular activation system, the limbic system and the orbitofrontal cortex. Various activation studies have demonstrated that ACh neurons which send their afferents to the temporal association cortex are not homogeneous from a physiological point of view; as a matter of fact, they have diverse rates and patterns of firing and discharge. For that reason, brain areas which are innervated by these ACh fibres possibly will be more controlled by single ACh neurons than other modulatory transmitters do. The transmitter ACh interacts with two main groups of receptors which are found in cortical target areas, namely with muscarinic and nicotinic receptors [Cooper et al., 2003; Klein et al., 2004; McNamara et al., 2004; Siegel et al., 2006].

It seems that cholinergic activity is greater in the left human hemisphere than in the right one. In particular, Amaducci et al. [1981] found that there is a greater choline acetyltransferase (ChAT) activity in the left human temporal lobe than in the right one. Glick et al. [1982] reported a greater ChAT activity in the left globus pallidus than in the right one. Moreover, Hutsler and Gazzaniga [1996] reported that the density and distribution of ACh containing axons and pyramidal cells differ methodically in the left posterior brain regions. In fact, they reported that there is a high density of acetyl-cholineesterase (AChE) containing axons inside the primary auditory cortex, whereas pyramidal cells are principally not present there. On the contrary, the putative language regions of the posterior cortex which are not localized within the primary auditory region have not only a high density of AChE containing axons, but also a high density of AChE containing pyramidal cells. Pyramidal cells of layer III of the left hemisphere which contain a high level of AChE are bigger than those found in the right hemisphere. This possibly will point to an increased ACh influence on left-sided output processes of speech and language areas. Furthermore, we know that the left temporal lobe is involved in the elaboration process of verbal memory, too; for that reason, finding high levels of ACh in that brain region suggests that ACh is also involved in the elaboration process of verbal memory. In conclusion, it can be remarked that ACh sensitive neurons are broadly scattered all over the brain, but cholinergic neurons are principally found in those neural networks which support speech and language, and therefore, the density of cholinergic neurons is higher in the left than in the right hemisphere [Klein et al., 2004; McNamara et al., 2004].

Serotonin

Serotonin, or 5-hydroxytryptamine (5-HT), is another central neurotransmitter, and neuronal cell bodies containing 5-HT are primarily found in isolated clusters of groups of cells placed along the midline of the brainstem. In spite of this, it was observed that their axons innervate almost every area of the CNS. In 1964, Dahlström and Fuxe noticed that the bulk of serotonergic cells are placed in the raphe nuclei. Furthermore, they described nine groups of serotonergic cell bodies (B_1-B_9) which match roughly with the raphe nuclei. But not all serotonergic cell bodies are localized within the raphe nuclei and not all the cell bodies found in the raphe nuclei are serotonergic. In fact, only 40-50% of the cell bodies found in the dorsal raphe are serotonergic, and 5-HT reactive cells were found in the area postrema and in the caudal locus ceruleus but also in and around the interpeduncular nucleus. The more caudal groups (B_1-B_4), which are localized from the mid pons to the caudal medulla, project to the medulla and spinal cord. The more rostral serotonergic cell groups (B_7-B_9), which are localized within the raphe dorsalis, raphe medianus, and raphe centralis superior, send their projections to the telencephalon and to the diencephalon (forebrain and other regions of the cerebral cortex). 5-HT neurons which are found in the raphe medianus and dorsalis are not only different in their electrophysiological characteristics and in their inhibition, but they also differ in the morphology and topographical organization of their axonal projections to the forebrain. The above-mentioned differences seem to be very important in understanding the role of 5-HT in normal brain function and in mental illness. There are two major ascending serotonergic pathways which send their projections from the midbrain raphe nuclei to the forebrain, i.e. the dorsal periventricular path and the ventral tegmental radiations which converge in the caudal hypothalamus. In the caudal hypothalamus, these two pathways meet the medial forebrain bundle. The dorsal and the median raphe nuclei give origin to two individual projections to forebrain regions, i.e. the median raphe sends its projections to the hippocampus, septum and hypothalamus. On the contrary, the dorsal raphe innervates the striatum. Both the dorsal and median raphe nuclei innervate the neocortex. For instance, the frontal cortex is innervated by the rostral and lateral subregions of the dorsal raphe nucleus. Moreover, it was seen that the raphe nuclei not only get input from the SN and VTA (DA), superior vestibular nucleus (ACh), LC (NE), nucleus prepositus hypoglossi and nucleus of the solitary tract (E), but also from the hypothalamus, cortex and limbic forebrain structures [Cooper et al., 2003; Siegel et al., 2006].

The neurotransmitter 5-HT is mainly stored in vesicles and released into the synaptic cleft through exocytosis. Its release is partly controlled by the firing rate of serotonergic neurons which are localized in the raphe nuclei. As a matter of fact, an increase in raphe cell firing augments the release of 5-HT in terminal fields. But if there is a decrease in raphe cell firing there is also a decrease in the release of 5-HT. For that reason, drugs which modify the firing rate of serotonergic neurons modify the release of 5-HT, too [Cooper et al., 2003; Siegel et al., 2006].

The neurotransmitter 5-HT is involved in almost every type of behavior (appetitive, emotional, motoric, cognitive and autonomic), but at the present time, we still do not know if 5-HT influences such behaviors explicitly or if it influences these types of behavior just by coordinating the activity of the nervous system. It was noticed that an alteration of the 5-HT system can cause particular modifications in the various types of behavior. In fact, there are some neuroactive drugs which interact with the serotonergic neurons and with their receptors, and which are used for treating particular disorders, such as depression, anxiety, and schizophrenia. Therefore, it can be pointed out that 5-HT supervises many forms of behavior and many different physiological processes [Cooper et al., 2003; Siegel et al., 2006].

Chapter 4

DEFINITION OF FLUENCY

In 1908, after having analyzed the quality of the speech production of aphasic patients, Carl Wernicke introduced the concept of "fluent" and "non-fluent" aphasia. This classification is still in use today. These two terms cannot be used according to their literal meaning, as the discrimination between fluent and non-fluent output is made on the basis not of a single dimension but of multiple dimensions of verbal production. None of which can be used alone for making a correct diagnosis of fluent and non-fluent aphasia. Fluent speech and non-fluent speech are the two extremes of a continuum and not two distinct categories. Moreover, fluency is not to be confused with the aberrant rhythm patterns typical of dysfluent speech; in other words, it is not to be confused with stuttering [Nadeau et al., 2000; Basso, 2005].

In order to evaluate the fluency of an aphasic subject in the best way possible, the examiner has to conduct an open dialogue with the patient and pay attention to the way in which he speaks. Not only the type of mistakes which the patient makes but also the adequacy of what he says are important elements which can be used for making a better diagnosis. But these elements should be analyzed later on after having ascertained whether the patient is fluent or not. There are some particular features of the spontaneous oral production which consent to make a non-controversial diagnosis [Nadeau et al., 2000; Basso, 2005].

Patients with agrammatism or verbal apraxia[3] are classified as non-fluent aphasics, but agrammatism is rather rare and verbal apraxia[4] is difficult to

---

[3] In the past, terms such as anarthria, articulatory difficulty and cortical dysarthria were used for referring to verbal apraxia.

diagnose. Aphasic patients who are affected by verbal apraxia have an alteration of the automatized articulation; the oral production is not only hindered and slowed down, but also characterized by a continuous search for the correct articulation point [Nadeau et al., 2000 Basso, 2005].

According to Albert et al. [1981], the fluency of an aphasic patient's verbal output can reflect function along a number of dimensions, including melody and prosody, phrase length, articulation agility, grammatical form, semantic access, presence of paraphasiae, and anomia. Each of these elements should be considered in determining the causes of a patient's loss of fluency and in defining treatment approaches. Nevertheless, it is rather rare that all these criteria are taken into consideration; the criterion which seems to be the most suitable one for making a correct distinction between fluent and non-fluent aphasia, if there is an absence of agrammatism and verbal apraxia is the phrase length. It was suggested that the presence of even one sentence of six words every ten sentences is enough to make a correct diagnosis of fluent aphasia; patients who are non-fluent do not speak much and use short sentences with no more than three words per sentence. While according to Nadeau et al. [2000], the dimensions of spoken language that allow a correct distinction between fluent and non-fluent aphasia are the quantity of speech (rate[5], phrase length, and thematic elaboration/communicative intent), articulatory agility, melody/prosody, and adequacy, and variety of grammatical form/syntax.

In general, there are three types of aphasias which are associated with non-fluent aphasia, namely Broca's aphasia, transcortical motor aphasia, and global aphasia; whereas Wernicke's aphasia, conduction aphasia, transcortical sensory aphasia and anomic aphasia are associated with fluent aphasia [Basso, 2005]. Therefore, it can be said that fluent aphasic speech is caused by a posterior lesion, and in general, this form of aphasia is associated with normal or excessive rate, normal phrase length, rhythm, melody, and articulated agility.

---

[4] Verbal apraxia is easy to recognize if the patient is affected by a severe form of verbal apraxia, whereas a mild form of verbal apraxia is rather difficult to recognize and is often mistaken for phonemic paraphasiae.

[5] It was measured that the speaking rate in conversational speech by normal adults ranges from 100 to 175 words per minute; and in aphasic subjects between 12 and 175 words per minute. Subjects with a speech rate below 50 words per minute are classified as distinctly subnormal, whereas subjects with a speech rate between 51 and 149 words per minute are considered normal [Nadeau et al., 2000].

On the contrary, non-fluent aphasia speech is caused by an anterior lesion and is associated with slow rate, reduced phrase length, abnormal intentional contour, effortful articulation, and simplified syntax and/or absent grammar [Nadeau et al., 2000]. Moreover, it must be pointed out that verbal fluency impairments can be also seen in non-aphasic patients who are affected by different types of frontal pathology [Amunts et al., 2004].

Chapter 5

NEUROPHARMACOLOGY OF
VERBAL FLUENCY, SPEECH,
AND LANGUAGE

Even though the neurochemistry of language and the neuropharmacology of speech and language disorders are two disciplines of cognitive neuroscience which are still in their infancy, in the 1950s, Luria proposed to use anticholinesterase drugs for treatment of aphasia [de Boissezon et al., 2007]. As already seen, many cortical and subcortical brain regions and polysynaptic pathways not only of the left but also of the right hemisphere are involved in the elaboration of the various complex neuronal and linguistic processes which are fundamental for our ability to speak and perceive language. Every single neuronal process executed by our brain is mediated by particular neurotransmitters; therefore, it is very likely that even cognitive processes, such as speech and language, are mediated by those neurotransmitters. In consequence, many drugs used in clinical practice, also with very different pharmacological action, may affect the complex neuroanatomical/biochemical network regulating speech and language and thus influence verbal fluency and other linguistic abilities. The implicated drugs include the old and new antiepileptic agents, neuroleptics, dopaminergic drugs, anticholinesterase drugs, β-blockers, antidepressants, benzodiazepines, and stimulant agents, such as cocaine and methylphenidate.

Today, it is clear that aphasia is caused by damage to the cortical and subcortical neuronal tissue and network which are involved in speech and language. Even in our days, research keeps on assessing and associating language function and lesion localization. Correct lesion localization is not only crucial for making a precise diagnosis of aphasia, but also for making a correct prognosis for recovery and for administering an adequate speech and language therapy. In addition, the study of spontaneous speech and language recovery makes it easier to understand those brain mechanisms which underlie aphasia. It has been seen that speech and language recovery is influenced by many different factors. Up to now, various efforts have been made to explain the recovery of speech and language after stroke. At the moment, there are two main hypotheses. On the one hand, it is believed that the right hemisphere takes up language functions and on the other, that there is greater activation of the residual neuronal cells of the left hemisphere. Neurofunctional data has shown that both hypotheses seem to be very plausible. In order to develop new and efficient therapies, in particular pharmacological ones, it is very important to understand what happens at the cellular and biochemical level when the brain tissue is damaged by a pathological event/process. There are various pathological events or processes which can cause aphasia, and the most important are ischemic stroke involving the left middle cerebral artery, traumatic brain injury, tumours, focal infections, and focal lobar degeneration. All these pathological processes are characterized by disruption of the blood-brain barrier. The disruption of the blood-brain barrier sets free a fast and complex cascade of biochemical events which cause damage to the neuronal brain tissue. For instance, an ischemic event induces the release of excitotoxic neurotransmitters, such as glutamate. These excitotoxic neurotransmitters are directly released from neurons and from glial cells, and they bind to receptors, such as NMDA, AMPA, and kainate, which in turn, induce the release of calcium. The calcium release causes the entry into the brain of sodium which increases the volume of intracellular water, and which in turn, induces neuronal swelling and membrane disruption. These fast and complex biochemical processes lead to cell death which has its greatest extent at the core and is less present in the surrounding tissue (penumbra). But if there is hyperglycemia, too, the concentration of lactic acid augments. The increase in lactic acid causes an enlargement of the core area of damage. For that reason, the chances of survival of the penumbral cells diminish, and this leads to bad clinical outcomes. Moreover, there is also the release of free radicals during the initial phases of an ischemic process. Free radicals destroy the fatty acids which form the cell membrane through a process called lipid peroxidation causing the death of neurons and glial cells. The dying neurons and glial cells activate macrophage scavenger cells. These processes of cell destruction can go on for weeks or months, and, therefore, they not only cause immediate cell death, but also secondary cell destruction. The neurons and glial cells which lie in close proximity to the destroyed tissue and which were not destroyed by the destructive cascade will remain weak forever. In conclusion, it can be said that if we understand the biochemical mechanisms which underlie these destructive processes, we will be able to use particular drugs which could stop the process of cell destruction [Klein et al., 2004].

Clinical studies have reported that there are cases in which the patient has an almost complete spontaneous recovery of speech and language. Today, we know that there are many different neuronal mechanisms which are involved in spontaneous recovery, for instance the cerebral area "A" is replaced by the cerebral area "B" (vicariance), an area of the brain which is generally not implicated in the processing of a particular task suddenly processes that task (functional substitution) and distant brain regions, which were initially suppressed, regain function (release from diaschisis). Research in molecular biology has shown that various biomolecular processes, such as regeneration of damaged cells and sprouting from non-damaged collateral cells are involved in recovery. These biomolecular processes are mediated by various neurotrophic factors, which are particular proteins, for instance the nerve growth factor (NGF). It was seen that NGF promotes nerve growth and leads the neurons to their target. Moreover, it is supposed that particular proteins, the so-called healing factors located at the site of lesion boost the process of regeneration and repair, while cell adhesion molecules which are found outside the site of lesion assist neurons in finding their target. In addition, it was observed that also glial cells stimulate the release of trophic factors which promote recovery. But trophic factors released by glial cells are involved in scar production, too, which hinder the recovery of neurons. So a further target of neuroscientific research is that of improving those mechanisms which are involved in brain repair through the specific use of particular drugs [Klein et al., 2004].

In conclusion, it has to be pointed out that further research is needed in order to find old or new molecules which could replace the neurotransmitters lost in cell death, antagonize the toxic substances produced during cell death, reduce the release of excitotoxic substances, block the release of calcium, introduce antioxidants, and re-establish normal blood flow [Klein et al., 2004].

What follows is a detailed overview of those drugs which are utilized to treat aphasia and of those which influence verbal fluency and other linguistic abilities either in a positive or negative way (Table 2).

Agents Which Increase Cerebral Perfusion

It has been reported that patients who were treated with thrombolytic drugs sometimes had a complete revascularization of those areas which had been damaged by an ischemic process. But after having analyzed the patients' recovery pattern more carefully; it has to be pointed out that the administration of thrombolytic agents leads to a partial functional restoring in the following days and weeks and not to a complete one. In general, the main positive effect of thrombolytic agents is that of alleviating the ischemic penumbra [de Boissezon et al., 2007].

Hillis and colleagues [2001] [de Boissezon et al., 2007] demonstrated that an increase of blood pressure which takes place immediately after the critical post onset period is very likely to restore functions in those cortical areas which are located in the vicinity of the core ischemic area and which are therefore poorly perfused. Hillis and colleagues studied six aphasic patients by means of perfusion weighted magnetic resonance imaging. Their language functions were tested every day over the first eight post-stroke days. Blood pressure was increased through NaCl perfusion or by means of an intravenous injection of the α_1-sympathomimetic agonist phenylephrine, followed by a per os treatment with salt, fludrocortisone, or midodrine. The increase of blood pressure facilitated cortical perfusion in five patients who had a left posterior temporal hypoperfusion for the most part in Brodmann's area 22. The neurolinguistic investigation revealed an improvement in naming and comprehension. While in another patient, the increase of blood pressure enhanced blood perfusion in the left inferior temporal cortex, i.e. in Brodmann's area 37. In this case, the neurolinguistic examination revealed an improvement in naming, but not in comprehension.

In another study, Hillis and colleagues [2004] [de Boissezon et al., 2007] demonstrated that there seems to be a tight relationship between cortical hypoperfusion in the classical language areas and aphasia typology. Hillis and colleagues studied 24 patients who were in the acute stroke phase, and they observed that in two patients the cortical revascularisation led to the complete disappearance of the aphasic symptoms.

The increase of blood pressure by means of particular drugs seems to have some beneficial effects on language deficits, in particular in those patients who are in the acute phase of stroke [de Boissezon et al., 2007]. But, according to us, further studies are needed in order to understand the mechanisms which are involved in the above-mentioned processes.

Pharmacological class	Drug	Neurotransmitter System	Effect
Cholinergic agents			
	Piracetam	Acetylcholine	Piracetam improves the function of the neurotransmitter acetylcholine via muscarinic cholinergic receptors.
	Aniracetam	Acetylcholine	Aniracetam has a direct cholinergic effect via release of acetylcholine.
	Bifemelane	Acetylcholine	Bifemelane acts through muscarinic acetylcholine receptors.
Antipsychotic agents			
	Haloperidol	Dopamine	Antagonist (Neuroleptics have a high affinity for dopamine receptors, in particular for D_2 dopamine receptors. They block the meso-limbic D_2 dopamine receptors, as well as those found in the nucleus accumbens, in the stria terminalis and in the striatum, and inactivate the dopaminergic neurons of the substantia nigra. The initial response to the administration of neuroleptics is the blockade of D_2 dopamine receptors and an increase of forebrain dopamine turnover, and what follows then is a decrease of dopamine activity. Moreover, haloperidol has a significant α_1-adrenergic receptor antagonist activity.)
Atypical antipsychotic agents			
	Clozapine	Dopamine Serotonin	Clozapine is an antagonist of D_1 and D_2 dopamine receptors, but it has a greater antagonistic property for D_3 and D_4 dopamine receptors.
		Acetylcholine Norepinephrine	Clozapine is also an antagonist of 5-HT_{2A} and 5-HT_{2C} serotonin receptors. Moreover, it has anticholinergic and antiadrenergic properties; and it has a greater specificity for mesolimbic dopaminergic neurons, while the nigrostriatal dopaminergic neurons are spared.
		Dopamine Serotonin	Risperidone is an antagonist of D_2 dopamine receptors and of 5-HT_{2A} serotonin receptors. Moreover, it is an antagonist of α_1 and α_2 adrenergic receptors.
	Risperidone	Norepinephrine	

Table 2. (Continued).

Pharmacological class	Drug	Neurotransmitter System	Effect
Calcium channel blockers			
	Nilvadipine	Calcium channel	Nilvadipine blocks the L-type calcium channels in vascular muscle cells.
Antidepressants			
	Fluoxetine	Serotonin	Selective serotonin reuptake inhibitor (SSRI)
	Fluvoxamine	Serotonin	Selective serotonin reuptake inhibitor (SSRI)
	Paroxetine	Serotonin	Selective serotonin reuptake inhibitor (SSRI)
	Sertraline	Serotonin	Selective serotonin reuptake inhibitor (SSRI)
	Selegiline	Dopamine	Selegiline is an irreversible inhibitor of monoamine oxidase (MAO) B.
		Norepinephrine Serotonin	Selegiline is used in the early stages of Parkinson's disease as it strengthens the effects of dopamine. Selegiline is also used as an antidepressant, i.e. high doses of selegiline can inhibit MAO-A.
	Tranylcypromine	Norepinephrine Serotonin Dopamine	Tranylcypromine is a reversible inhibitor of MAO-A and MAO-B. It increases the concentration of dopamine, serotonin and norepinephrine.
	Moclobemide	Norepinephrine Serotonin Dopamine	Moclobemide is a reversible inhibitor of MAO-A, and it has a low affinity for cholinergic, H_1-histaminergic or α_1-adrenergic receptors.
Atypical antidepressants			
	Trazodone	Serotonin	Trazodone is a weak selective serotonin reuptake inhibitor, and it is an antagonist of $5\text{-}HT_{1A}$, $5\text{-}HT_{1C}$ and $5\text{-}HT_2$ serotonin receptors. Its active metabolite, mCPP, is a powerful agonist of serotonin. Trazodone is a mixed agonist-antagonist of serotonin. It is also a quite powerful antagonist of postsynaptic α_1-adrenergic receptors.

Pharmacological class	Drug	Neurotransmitter System	Effect
Anxiolytic agents			
	Buspirone	Serotonin	Buspirone is an agonist of presynaptic 5-HT$_{1A}$ serotonin receptors (localized in the dorsal nucleus of the raphe) which cause an inhibition of the neuronal firing and a decrease of the synthesis of serotonin. Buspirone is also a partial agonist of postsynaptic 5-HT$_{1A}$ serotonin receptors which are localized in the hippocampus and in the cortex. If there is an excess of functional serotonin, buspirone behaves like an antagonist, but on the contrary if there is a deficit of serotonin, it behaves like an agonist.
	Meprobamate	GABA	Meprobamate acts through GABA, even if it does not bind to specific GABA receptors.
β-blockers			
	Propranolol	Norepinephrine (β$_1$ and β$_2$)	Propranolol is a non-selective antagonist of β$_1$ and β$_2$ adrenergic receptors.
Hypnotics (imidazopiridines)			
	Zolpidem	GABA	Zolpidem is a selective agonist of the ω$_1$ site of GABA$_A$ receptors.

Dopaminergic Agents

Until now, many drugs were used for treating language impairment in aphasic patients. But in modern times, the first drugs which were used for treating speech and language disorder in aphasic patients were dopaminergic drugs, such as the dopamine agonist bromocriptine, as it is believed that such substances are able to influence the language output pathways [de Boissezon et al., 2007; Klein et al., 2004]. Albert et al. [1988], Gupta and Mlcoch [1992], Sabe et al. [1992] [de Boissezon et al., 2007; Klein et al., 2004] used the dopamine agonist bromocriptine in an open-label trial to treat the language impairment in aphasic patients. They observed that the administration of bromocriptine caused an improvement of fluency, naming and hesitations in connected speech. It has been noticed that these improvements regarded disorders of language production, shortening verbal latency or reaction time for language response [Albert et al., 1988; Gupta & Mlcoch, 1992; Sabe et al., 1992; Gold et al., 2000; Raymer et al., 2001; Reed et al., 2004 cited in de Boissezon et al., 2007]. It must be highlighted that these improvements have been noticed in those aphasic patients who had a mild speech and language impairment due to subcortical lesions and in those who are affected by a moderate transcortical motor aphasia. Albert et al. [1988] studied and analyzed the alterations of speech fluency of aphasic patients because they were of the opinion that the same lack of neurotransmitters which causes hesitancies and bradykinesia in Parkinson's disease could cause the bradykinesia of speech in patients with transcortical motor aphasia. Various studies showed that the midbrain dopaminergic system not only sends its projections to medial frontal areas (mesocortical system) but also to the caudate and putamen (nigrostriatal system) [Albert et al., 1988]. It is known that lesions of the left medial frontal regions can cause a transcortical motor aphasia, and for that reason Albert and colleagues supposed that some particular characteristics which are typical of transcortical motor aphasia could be caused by the interruption of the mesocortical projection [Albert et al., 1988]. But other research groups, such as Gupta et al. [1995], Sabe et al. [1995], Reed et al. [2004] [de Boissezon et al., 2007] and Ashtary et al. [2005] which used bromocriptine in randomized, placebo-controlled studies did not confirm the observations made by Albert and colleagues in the study of 1988 [de Boissezon et al., 2007]. Bragoni et al. [2000] administered bromocriptine in combination with speech therapy in order to enhance recovery in stable chronic non-fluent aphasic patients. They reported that the administration of high doses of bromocriptine combined with speech therapy had some beneficial effects; in fact, according to them, their patients showed a significant improvement in language during treatment [Bragoni et al., 2000]. But if the research protocol and the obtained results are analyzed more carefully, this study will inevitably raise various doubts. The treatment order was fixed in all cases, and the study was divided into five phases. It is worth mentioning that at the end of the second phase (placebo associated with speech therapy) there was only a significant improvement in dictation [Bragoni et al., 2000; de Boissezon et al., 2007]. While at the end of the third phase (bromocriptine associated with speech therapy), there was a decrease in verbal latency and an improvement in dictation and in reading-comprehension when compared with baseline values [Bragoni et al., 2000]. According to de Boissezon and colleagues [2007], these improvements could be caused by the administration of bromocriptine associated with speech therapy or by the four month-long speech therapy. Moreover, it is important to point out that the scores of the various language tests decreased after the fourth phase (bromocriptine alone), but the verbal latency and reading-comprehension scores turned out to be still significantly high [de Boissezon et al., 2007]. At the end of the fifth phase, i.e. the wash-out phase, the scores regarding the verbal latency task were not anymore significantly high [Bragoni et al., 2000; de Boissezon et al., 2007].

In conclusion, it must be highlighted that dopaminergic agents, such as bromocriptine, can cause various side effects which range from dizziness, drowsiness, and fainting (common side effects) to nausea, vomiting, gastrointestinal upset, atrial fibrillation, and visual hallucinations (less-common side effects) [Klein et al., 2004; Bragoni et al., 2000]. Furthermore, it seems that the administration of dopaminergic agents, such as bromocriptine does not significantly improve the speech and language deficits of aphasic patients, and the first encouraging studies appear to be quite anecdotic [de Boissezon et al., 2007].

Amphetamines

Results from animal studies suggest that the administration of amphetamines associated with training can improve the recovery from stroke-induced deficits [Feeney et al., 1982; Feeney et al., 1987 cited in de Boissezon et al., 2007] [Martinsson et al., 2004], for instance it has been observed that the administration of dextroaphetamine increased neural sprouting and synaptogenesis [Goldstein et al., 1990 cited in de Boissezon et al., 2007]. In addition, it has been reported that the functional recovery was greater when amphetamines were administered in combination with practice or training [de Boissezon et al., 2007], but the positive effects caused by the combination of drug therapy with training seem to rely on the time window in which drug therapy and training are administered; for instance, a treatment which takes place too early seems to have deleterious effects [Kozlowski et al., 1996 cited in de Boissezon et al., 2007], whereas there are no positive effects if the treatment takes place too late [Feeney et al., 1985 cited in de Boissezon et al., 2007].

In 2001, Walker-Batson and colleagues [de Boissezon et al., 2007] published an important study on the effects of dexamphetamine treatment of aphasia. They studied 21 patients in a randomized, placebo-controlled study, and all patients were at subacute stroke stage and had nonhemorrhagic strokes with moderate to severe aphasia [Klein et al., 2004; de Boissezon et al., 2007]. This study lasted five weeks, and the administration of either dexamphetamine or placebo happened 30 minutes before speech therapy (ten 1-hour sessions of speech therapy). The patients who received the active drug had a faster rate of aphasia recovery than those who received the placebo. Therefore, one week after the completion of the treatment, the group which received dexamphetamine had better language performances than the placebo group. Walker-Batson and colleagues [2001] used a well-designed research protocol for their study, and the obtained results revealed that dexamphetamine could have some positive effects on language recovery [de Boissezon et al., 2007]. But the study suffers potential bias inasmuch as dexamphetamine was administered during an active period of spontaneous recovery [Klein et al., 2004].

Another important study which investigated the effects of dexamphetamine combined with standard naming therapy was done by Whiting et al. in 2007. They looked at two patients in a double-blind, placebo-controlled, multiple base-line, crossover study. Both patients were in the chronic stage of stroke recovery. Whiting et al. [2007] demonstrated that dexamphetamine paired with combined semantic and phonological therapy could be helpful for the treatment of naming disorders in chronic aphasia. These results are in clear contrast with those which suggest that dexamphetamine may improve language recovery in patients at subacute stroke stage, but not in patients who are in the chronic stage of stroke recovery [Whiting et al., 2007; de Boissezon et al., 2007]. In fact, it is believed that amphetamines, in particular dexamphetamine have some neuromodulatory effects on brain plasticity only during the early recovery phase [Whiting et al., 2007; de Boissezon et al., 2007]. But, these results indicate that the administration of amphetamines combined with speech therapy could have some positive effects in patients with a chronic aphasia, too [Whiting et al., 2007]. The results reported in this study are interesting and promising, but the number of patients studied by Whiting and colleagues is too small, and, therefore, the results obtained in this study are not very significant.

Up to now, only few studies regarding the effects of dexamphetamine in aphasic patients have been done, and therefore further clinical trials involving more patients are required [Whiting et al., 2007; de Boissezon et al., 2007]. Moreover, additional studies are needed in order to understand whether amphetamines are more helpful in the acute or post-stroke phase [Whiting et al., 2007]. Hemiplegic patients treated with amphetamines reported improvements of motor deficit. This demonstrates that amphetamines improve not only cognitive deficits but also motor deficits [Walker-Batson et al., 1995 cited in de Boissezon et al., 2007]. According to Martinsson and colleagues [2004], amphetamines should not be used in clinical practice as the mortality rate is higher in patients treated with amphetamines than in those treated with placebo.

Serotonin

Early experimental studies demonstrated that the use of serotonergic agents improved post-stroke motor deficits not only in animals but also in human beings, and for that reason various research groups wanted to verify whether serotonergic drugs were able to improve aphasia or not [de Boissezon et al., 2007]. The selective serotonin reuptake inhibitors (SSRI), such as fluoxetine, fluvoxamine, sertraline, and paroxetine are the most used and studied serotonergic agents in humans [Klein et al., 2004; de Boissezon et al., 2007].

Loubinox and colleagues [de Boissezon et al., 2007] studied eight patients with motor hemiplegia, and they demonstrated through the use of fMRI that fluoxetine overactivates the primary motor cortex improving motor performance. In another study, Loubinox et al. [2005] [de Boissezon et al., 2007] studied the effects of paroxetine in healthy subjects. They observed that a chronic treatment with paroxetine had beneficial effects on some particular aspects of motor performance, but it also reduced fMRI activation in some of those brain areas which form the motor system. In particular, it has been noticed that paroxetine decreased fMRI activation in the sensory motor cortex.

Tanaka et al. [2004] [de Boissezon et al., 2007] studied the effects of fluvoxamine in ten aphasic patients in a double-blind, crossover, randomized study. The treatment with fluvoxamine lasted four weeks, and Tanaka and colleagues reported improvements in mood and naming in fluent aphasic patients [Klein et al., 2004; de Boissezon et al., 2007].

Peran et al. [2004] [de Boissezon et al., 2007] studied the effects of paroxetine on verb production in healthy subjects through the use of fMRI. They observed that if verb-related semantic representations were associated with oral production then the left parietal cortex was modulated in a particular way by paroxetine, but if verb-related semantic representations were associated with mental stimulation of action, then the left parietal cortex was modulated in a different way.

Additional studies are required in order to understand and verify the effects of serotonergic agents in aphasic patients [de Boissezon et al., 2007].

Cholinergic Drugs

Acetylcholine functions as a cortical modulator which is involved in task-related plasticity and long-term potentiation, and for that reason it is indispensable for learning, memory, language and attention. Cholinergic pathways can be damaged or even destroyed by a cerebrovascular accident (CVA), for instance a CVA which hits the left hemisphere and which involves the insulo-opercular cortex, white matter tracts or the mesial frontoparietal cortex will probably damage the cholinergic pathways, which are involved in language processing [Berthier et al., 2006].

The acetylcholinesterase inhibitors, such as ameridin, physostigmine, galantamine, rivastigmine, and donepezil were and/or are used against cognitive impairment in patients affected by Alzheimer's disease [Klein et al., 2004; de Boissezon et al., 2007]. Various scientists assume that acetylcholinesterase inhibitors and other cholinergic agents can have some beneficial effects in aphasic patients as these drugs modulate the cholinergic pathway, and for that reason it is assumed that they can improve lexical-semantic processes and verbal memory [de Boissezon et al., 2007]. Therefore, it can be hypothesised that these drugs can improve deficits in comprehension in patients with temporal lesions [de Boissezon et al., 2007].

Various studies have been published which investigated the effects of cholinergic agents in aphasic patients. Luria [1970] [Klein et al., 2004] investigated the effects of galantamine in aphasic patients. He reported that the patients who received galantamine had improvements in articulation, paraphasias, naming, comprehension, and fluency.

Tanaka et al. [1997] [Klein et al., 2004] studied the effects of bifemelane in four patients with left temporal lobe lesions in a placebo-controlled study. They reported that the administration of bifemelane combined with speech therapy had some beneficial effects. In fact, according to them, the two patients who received bifemelane combined with speech therapy had greater improvement in auditory comprehension, animal naming and confrontation naming than those who received speech therapy without drug therapy.

In another study Tanaka et al. [2001] [de Boissezon et al., 2007] investigated the effects of aniracetam in eight patients with Wernicke's aphasia. They used nivaldipine as placebo, and the study lasted four weeks. They observed that the administration of aniracetam caused a significant improvement in naming but not in verbal memory.

Berthier et al. [2003] [de Boissezon et al., 2007] studied the effects of donepezil in eleven chronic aphasic patients. The study lasted 16 weeks, and they used the same protocol as in Alzheimer's disease, i.e. 5mg/day for four weeks and then 10mg/day. Berthier and colleagues reported significant improvements after four weeks of treatment, and these improvements were even more significant after sixteen weeks. Berthier and colleagues observed significant improvements in repetition, comprehension, phonetic discrimination and naming, but these improvements vanished after drug withdrawal. This indicates that donepezil acts in a direct way [de Boissezon et al., 2007].

In another study, Berthier et al. [2006] investigated the effects of donepezil in twenty-six chronic post-stroke aphasic patients in a randomized, placebo-controlled, double-blind parallel trial. The study lasted 20 weeks (4 weeks titration, 12 weeks maintenance and 4 weeks wash-out), and they used the same protocol as in Alzheimer's disease, i.e. 5mg/day of donepezil or placebo for four weeks and then 10mg/day of donepezil or placebo for twelve weeks. In this study Berthier and colleagues obtained similar results as in the previous study [Berthier et al., 2003 cited in de Boissezon at al., 2007], i.e. they observed significant improvements after four weeks of treatment with donepezil, and these improvements were even more significant after sixteen weeks. But, these improvements almost vanished after drug withdrawal. This suggests that donepezil enhances language and communication performance only when it is being taken [Berthier et al., 2006].

In conclusion, it has to be pointed out that additional placebo-controlled randomized studies are needed in order to confirm the above mentioned results regarding the effects of acetylcholinesterase inhibitors on phonological input/output processes and on lexical-semantic processes [de Boissezon et al., 2007].

Piracetam

Piracetam is a nootropic agent and a GABA derivate, which acts at the level of the cell membrane to which it binds [Huber, 1999]. It promotes cholinergic and glutamatergic neurotransmission [Huber, 1999; Klein et al., 2004; de Boissezon et al., 2007]; and it is assumed that piracetam reduces capillary vasospasm and thrombosis, and increases the cell membrane flexibility and oxygen extraction [Huber, 1999; de Boissezon et al., 2007]. Furthermore, experimental placebo-controlled studies in animals and healthy human beings revealed that piracetam improved learning and memory performance [Huber, 1999; de Boissezon et al., 2007].

Up to now various research groups studied the effects of piracetam in aphasic patients. Enderby et al. [1994], Huber et al. [1997], Kessler et al. [2000], Orgogozo [1999], and Szelies et al. [2001] [de Boissezon et al., 2007] investigated the effects of piracetam in aphasic patients in placebo-controlled studies, and they all reported that the patients who were treated with piracetam had a slight improvement in language.

Orgogozo [1999] [de Boissezon et al., 2007] looked at 373 aphasic patients who were treated with piracetam some hours after the onset of the CVA. Many patients who were treated with piracetam had a complete recovery from aphasia twelve weeks after the onset of the CVA. But this study suffers potential bias inasmuch as aphasia was not investigated in details, i.e. Orgogozo used the Frenchay screening aphasia test which is not suitable for such a study [de Boissezon et al., 2007].

Kessler et al. [2000] [Klein et al., 2004; de Boissezon et al., 2007] investigated the effects of piracetam in twenty-four aphasic patients in a randomized, placebo-controlled trial. The patients studied by this research group were treated with piracetam or placebo two weeks after the onset of the CVA. Furthermore, the language assessment (Aachen aphasia test) was performed in combination with PET measurements in an activation experiment (word repetition versus resting state). According to Kessler and colleagues, the patients who were treated with the active drug improved in seven sub-scores of the Aachen aphasia test, whereas those who received the placebo showed improvements in three sub-scores. The PET study revealed improvement in cerebral blood flow in the left superior temporal and inferior frontal regions which was greater in the patients treated with piracetam than in those who received the placebo [Klein et al., 2004; de Boissezon et al., 2007]. But this study suffers potential bias inasmuch as piracetam was administered during an active period of spontaneous recovery [Klein et al., 2004].

It has to be mentioned that piracetam is the most investigated pharmacological agent in aphasic patients, and all research groups reported that the patients treated with piracetam had a slight improvement in language, but additional double blind, multi centre, placebo-controlled studies are needed in order to confirm these results, and, therefore, its use in clinical practice should be avoided [de Boissezon et al., 2007].

Zolpidem

Zolpidem is a hypnotic agent and a selective agonist of the ω_1 site of GABA$_A$ receptors [Schatzberg & Nemeroff, 2001], and it has a short half-live [de Boissezon et al., 2007]. Cohen et al. [2004] [de Boissezon et al., 2007] studied the effects of zolpidem in a patient with a severe anterior aphasia. They reported that the patient had a noticeable improvement of speech fluency twenty minutes after the treatment with zolpidem. The single-photon emission computed tomography (SPECT) investigation revealed an augmentation of blood flow in Broca's area, in various areas of the left inferior frontal cortex which do not belong to Broca's area and in the left supra-marginal gyrus. However, the various mechanisms which are involved in the above mentioned processes remain still unclear. Clauss et al. [2000] [de Boissezon et al., 2007] investigated the effects of zolpidem in an aphasic patient, and the results described by Clauss and colleagues were similar to those described by Cohen and co-workers in the paper of 2004 [de Boissezon et al., 2007]. Additional studies are needed not only to understand the mechanisms which underlie these processes, but also to confirm these results [de Boissezon et al., 2007].

Amantadine

Amantadine is an antiviral agent, but it is also used for treating the typical symptoms of early Parkinson's patients. In fact, amantadine increases the release of dopamine and of other catecholamines from nerve terminals, but it also influences the acetylcholinergic and glutamatergic receptors. Amantadine has a preferential selectivity for central catecholaminergic neurons [Hardman et al., 2001; Schatzberg & Nemeroff, 2001]. Barrett and Eslinger [2007] investigated the effects of amantadine in four patients with transcortical motor aphasia in an open-label trial. They reported that the four patients who were treated with amantadine showed improvement in fluency (word generation), but at the end of the trial fluency was still below the normal range.

In conclusion, it has to be pointed out, that this study suffers potential bias inasmuch as amatadine was not administered in a double blind, placebo-controlled trial, and for that reason further studies are needed to confirm the above mentioned results. Moreover, it seems that the administration of amatadine does not significantly improve fluency.

Antiepileptic Agents

Levetiracetam is a highly effective novel antiepileptic drug which is similar to piracetam and which is used for treating focal epilepsies [Gomer et al., 2007]. Levetiracetam binds to the vesicular protein SV2A and influences the vesicular functions, thus modifying the release of synaptic glutamate and GABA [Schatzberg & Nemeroff, 2001; Katzung, 2007]. Up to now, only a studies regarding the cognitive effects of levetiracetam have been published [Piazzini et al., 2006].

Piazzini et al. [2006] studied the effects of levetiracetam in thirty-five patients with drug resistant partial epilepsy in a single-centre, add-on, open study. The neuropsychological test battery was administered before treatment with levetiracetam (baseline) and at the end of the treatment, i.e. seven weeks later. They compared the neuropsychological results of the patients treated with levetiracetam with those seen in a control group. Piazzini and co-workers reported that the patients treated with levetiracetam showed a significant improvement in attention and in oral fluency compared to controls.

Sechi et al. [2006] investigated the effects of levetiracetam in five patients with partial epilepsy and dis-fluent speech in a 9-week, open-label, prospective study. They administered levetiracetam combined with carbamazepine or phenytoin, and the fluency was assessed with the verbal fluency test at baseline and after 9 weeks. All patients treated with levetiracetam improved significantly in verbal fluency and in the speed of oral reading.

Topiramate is a highly effective novel antiepileptic drug with a half-live of about 20-30 hours which is used for treating partial-onset seizures, primary generalized tonic-clonic seizures, seizures associated with Lennox-Gastaut syndrome and juvenile myoclonic epilepsy [Meador et al., 2003; Gomer et al., 2007; Katzung, 2007]. Topiramate is a sulfamate-substituted monosaccharide, and its chemical structure is different from all other antiepileptic agents [Katzung, 2007]. Topiramate blocks voltage-dependent Na^+-channels, modulates high-voltage-activated Ca^{2+}-channels, increases the post-synaptic flow of chloride ions which is mediated by $GABA_A$ receptors (i.e. it potentiates GABAergic neuroinhibition) and decreases the activation of glutamate receptors which belong to the AMPA-kainate subtype [Schatzberg & Nemeroff, 2001; Meador et al., 2003; Gross-Tsur et al., 2004; Katzung, 2007]. Various clinical studies [Meador et al., 2003; Gross-Tsur et al., 2004; Gomer et al., 2007] demonstrated that topiramate has a variety of cognitive side effects which range from psychomotor slowing, memory and attentional problems to slow information processing and poor performance in verbal fluency tasks. These side effects have been observed both in patients with epilepsy and healthy subjects and suggest that topiramate may impair frontal lobe functions. In conclusion, it has to be mentioned that all authors reported relevant speech and language side effects [Meador et al., 2003; Gross-Tsur et al., 2004; Gomer et al., 2007].

Drugs Which Have Speech and Language Side Effects

There are some drugs which have speech and language side effects for instance, the anti-mitotic agent irinotecan which is used for treating metastatic colorectal carcinoma caused speech and language disorders, such as dysarthria or dysarthria followed by frank aphasia in three patients some minutes after infusion [Sevilla et al., 1999; Baz et al., 2001; De Marco et al., 2004 cited in de Boissezon et al., 2007].

Some psychotropic drugs, such as neuroleptics (e.g. haloperidol), thiazidics and tricyclic anti-depressants can also impair speech and language [Porch et al., 1985 cited in de Boissezon et al., 2007]. It has been reported that tricyclic anti-depressants may cause speech blockade, and, therefore, they impair verbal fluency [Klein et al., 2004].

Moreover, it has been reported that the anticholinergic drug scopolamine impairs working memory and the storage as well as the retrieval of verbal memory [Klein et al., 2004].

CLINICAL CASE

M.N. is a 32-year-old right-handed male with 13 years of school attendance. In summer 1995, M.N. was seriously injured through a bad car accident—he had a severe craniocerebral injury and multiple contusions all over his body. As M.N. went into a coma, he was put in intensive care in the City Hospital of Sassari. He came out of coma after three days, and afterwards, he was moved to the Hospital "Santa Corona" in Garvagnate Milanese where he underwent motor and cognitive rehabilitation. He stayed in the Hospital "Santa Corona" from the 13th July 1995 to the 30th October 1995.

M.N. came to our attention at the end of November 1995, and the anamnesis revealed that he was suffering from partial epileptic seizures which were most likely an after-effect of the previous craniocerebral injury. The neurological investigation revealed a mild right facial-brachial-crural hemiparesis, minimal signs of hypertonia at the right upper limb, a motor control deficit of the right limbs regarding the execution of fine movements and a slight sthenic deficit at the right inferior limb with a light hyperactivity of the patellar reflex. In addition, the right upper limb was adducted and flexed. The first informal dialogue with the patient showed that M.N. was affected by a light form of non-fluent dysphasia. M.N.'s speech and language disorder coincides with that observed in patients with damage to the subcortical structures and networks which are involved in the elaboration and processing of speech and language.

The magnetic resonance imaging (MRI) study revealed the presence of an irregular and non-homogeneous area of altered signal in the region of the left basal ganglia, small areas of hyperintensity involving the posterior arm of the internal capsule and the inferior posterior part of the lenticular nucleus, and a small area of hyperintense signal in the right inferior posterior thalamus.

It was decided to treat M.N.'s partial epileptic seizures with carbamazepine, 200mg three times a day. The patient had a good response to therapy, and as M.N. had not had any seizures since 1996, it was decided to stop antiepileptic medication beginning from March 1999.

The medical examination of the 14th January 2008 done in another neurological centre revealed that M.N. was in a state of "incipient depression", and it was decided to give him 100mg of topiramate twice a day in order to stabilize his mood. In March 2008, M.N. reported a serious worsening of his pre-existent, very mild speech and language disorder, and for that reason he was again seen in our neurological ward for further medical and neuro-psychological examination.

99mTc HM-PAO Brain SPECT

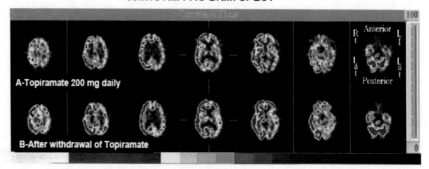

Figure 2. 99mTc HM-PAO brain SPECT: A: the patient has been taking topiramate 100mg twice a day for 3 months. A severe impairment of verbal fluency has been noticed. A severe reduction of cortical tracer uptake in the left brain hemisphere and focal areas of low uptake in the right temporal and parietal lobes are evident; B: about ten months after withdrawal of topiramate. The verbal fluency is still lightly impaired, but it improved considerably. The 99mTc HM-PAO uptake is globally improved, particularly in the right temporal and parietal lobes and in the left fronto-parietal and temporo-parietal cortical areas.

In March 2008, on topiramate therapy, M.N. underwent a first brain 99mTc HM-PAO SPECT investigation (figure 2 and figure 3), which revealed a severe reduction of cortical tracer uptake in the left brain hemisphere and focal areas of low uptake in the right temporal and parietal lobes.

We used the "Language Evaluation Test II"[6] by Ciurli, Marangolo and Basso [1996] to assess M.N.'s linguistic abilities. The first neurolinguistic investigation of the 13th March 2008 (figure 4) revealed a serious worsening of M.N.'s pre-existent speech and language disorder. M.N.'s oral output was characterized by very long pauses (four to five seconds) and by a severe dysprosody. The increase of the length of the pauses between one word and the other compromised the normal speech fluency. He spoke very slowly and with much difficulty. M.N. had such a severe alteration of normal speech rhythm, prosody and accentuation of words that he almost sounded as if he

---

[6] The "Language Evaluation Test II" evaluates the different aspects of oral and written language by means of the following tasks: 1) Verbal expression task (Description of a complex scene and Naming [nouns and verbs]); 2) Oral comprehension task (Comprehension of words, Comprehension of semantically related words and Comprehension of sentences); 3) Repetition of words, neologisms and sentences; 4) Writing task (Naming of nouns, Naming of verbs and Naming of a complex scene); 5) Reading comprehension task (Words, Semantically related words, and Sentences); 6) Reading aloud (Words, Sentences and Neologisms); 7) Dictation (Words, Sentences and Neologisms); 8) Coping (Words).

was stuttering. There were also some phonemic paraphasiae with the distortion of the phonemes, i.e. M.N. produced various phonemes which did not belong to the Italian language. In addition, there were also signs of agrammatism and anomia, for instance difficulty to recall words, in particular verbs, and for that reason he was not able to finish a sentence. In this case, he tried to rebuild the same sentence by using another verb. The sentences produced by M.N. were rather short and syntactically and grammatically poor. Moreover, M.N.'s handwriting tended to be very small, and sometimes there were signs of perseveration, too, i.e. there was the tendency to rewrite the same grapheme again and again. Thus, his handwriting was illegible most of the time. In conclusion, it can be said that M.N. was affected by a severe form of non-fluent dysphasia.

It has to be pointed out that, in this case, topiramate acted on an already compromised neuronal network, and for that reason it aggravated M.N.'s pre-existent speech and language disorder. We decided to interrupt the pharmacological treatment with topiramate after having realized that topiramate aggravated M.N.'s pre-existent speech and language disorder. Beginning from April 2008, we decreased 25mg of the topiramate dose every fortnight, so that we had a complete wash-out of topiramate approximately after sixteen weeks. We have noticed an improvement of M.N.'s speech and language abilities during and after the suspension of topiramate, and he got a complete stabilization of his speech and language disorder within three months.

M.N. underwent a second SPECT investigation (figure 2 and figure 3) in May 2009, i.e. approximately 10 months after withdrawal of topiramate. The 99mTc HM-PAO uptake was globally improved, particularly in the right temporal and parietal lobes and in the left fronto-parietal and temporo-parietal cortical areas.

The second neurolinguistic investigation of the 01st July 2009 (figure 5) revealed a speech and language disorder which coincides with that observed in patients with damage to the subcortical structures and networks which are involved in the elaboration and processing of speech and language. M.N.'s oral output was characterized by long pauses (approximately two/three seconds) and by a mild dysprosody. The increase of the length of the pauses between one word and the other compromised the normal speech fluency. There were still some phonemic paraphasiae with distortion of the phonemes. Furthermore, there were also some signs of agrammatism and anomia, for instance difficulty to recall words, in particular verbs, and for that reason he was not able to finish a sentence. In this case he tried to rebuild the same sentence by using another verb. The sentences produced by M.N. were rather short and syntactically and grammatically poor. M.N.'s **handwriting** improved considerably, so that it was within normal range. In conclusion, it can be said that M.N.'s verbal fluency is still lightly impaired, but it improved considerably. M.N. is affected by a mild form of non-fluent dysphasia.

Multi Threshold Volume: 67%

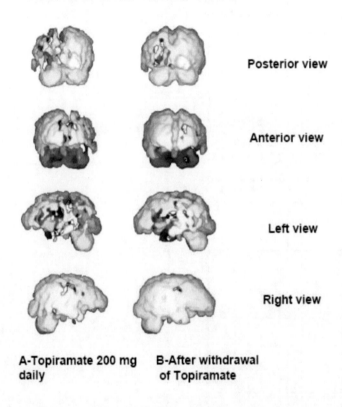

Figure 3. 99mTc HM-PAO brain SPECT: (A) at the 1° observation there was a severe reduction of cortical tracer uptake in the left brain hemisphere and focal areas of low uptake in the right temporal and parietal lobes. (B): About 10 months after drug wash-out, 99mTc HM-PAO uptake globally improved, particularly in the right temporal and parietal lobes and in the left fronto-parietal and temporo-parietal cortical areas.

Verbal expression task			Oral. Comp.		Repetition			Writing			Read. Com.		R. Aloud			Dict.			Copy
Nam. Fig.	Nam. Ns.	Nam. Vs.	P	PSA	F	P	N	F	Nam. Ns.	Nam. Vs	Nam.Fig.	P	PSA	F	P	N	F	P	N	F	Words

Figure 4. First "Language Evaluation Test II" (Nam. Fig.: Figure naming, Nam. Ns: Naming nouns, Nam. Vs.: Naming verbs, Oral. Comp.: Oral comprehension, Read. Comp.: Reading comprehension, R. aloud: Reading aloud, Dict.: Dictation).

Verbal expression task			Oral. Comp.			Repetition			Writing			Read. Com.			R. Aloud			Dict.			Copy
Nam. Fig.	Nam. Ns.	Nam. Vs.	P	PSA	F	P	N	F	Nam. Ns.	Nam. Vs	Nam. Fig.	P	PSA	F	P	N	F	P	N	F	Words

Figure 5. Second "Language Evaluation Test II" (Nam. Fig.: Figure naming, Nam. Ns: Naming nouns, Nam. Vs.: Naming verbs, Oral. Comp.: Oral comprehension, Read. Comp.: Reading comprehension, R. aloud: Reading aloud, Dict.: Dictation).

CONCLUSION

Many of the above-mentioned research studies have not reported significant speech and language improvements in patients who were treated with pharmacological agents alone for instance, aphasic patients who were treated with the dopaminergic agent bromocriptine showed no significant language improvements. In fact, these results do not encourage the regular use of drugs as a treatment for aphasia. Some beneficial effects have been reported when the pharmacological treatment for aphasia was associated with speech therapy. According to Small [1994], not many scientists were aware of this, and therefore the expectancies of most of the scientists were rather unrealistic. At the present time, we do not know if the improvements are ascribable to speech therapy alone or to the combination of drug therapy with speech therapy. According to Paradis [2004], speech therapy is focused whether consciously or unconsciously on metalinguistic knowledge[7]. In other words, speech therapists use techniques or strategies which are based on the use of explicit knowledge; for instance, a patient is treated by explicitly drawing his attention to the linguistic exercise in the same way as a second language learner is when he is learning his second language in school. The language improvements obtained by aphasic patients who receive speech therapy could

---

[7] Implicit linguistic competence (i.e. phonology, morphology, syntax and lexicon) is that form of knowledge which is deduced from an individuals' systematic verbal performance, but in general, the speakers are not aware of the existence of it. In other words, this particular competence is acquired in an unconscious way and stored implicitly; and therefore, it is used involuntarily. Metalinguistic knowledge is that form of knowledge of which individuals are conscious, i.e. the conscious knowledge of language facts (form, structure and rules of a language). This form of knowledge is consciously learned and can be recalled on demand in a conscious way and is stored in the declarative memory system [Paradis, 2004].

also be explained through the threshold hypothesis, according to which, an item is activated as soon as a sufficient quantity of positive neural impulses have reached its neural substrate. The activation threshold is the quantity of positive impulses which are needed for the activation of the item. Every time a particular item is activated, its activation threshold is lowered, and for that reason, fewer neural impulses are needed to reactivate that particular item. So, according to the threshold hypothesis, it is difficult to activate an item which is not stimulated enough as its activation threshold is higher than that of an item which is continuously stimulated. An item which is easily activated needs fewer resources to be reactivated. For that reason, an intensive use and/or intensive and prolonged exposure to a particular language lowers the activation threshold for that language. The continuous exercise through speech therapy lowers the activation threshold for a particular language, and for that reason the patient who receives speech therapy shows language improvements [Paradis, 2004].

Only very view pharmacological agents showed some beneficial effects for instance, it seems that piracetam and amphetamines increase cerebral plasticity which improves functional recovery [Klein et al., 2004; de Boissezon et al., 2007]. But, if drug therapy takes place too early, i.e. in the acute stroke phase, then we do not know if the observed improvements are ascribable to pharmacological treatment or to spontaneous recovery [Klein et al., 2004]. In general, it is quite difficult to separate improvements due to spontaneous recovery from those obtained through drug therapy [Klein et al., 2004]. Moreover, various research groups [de Boissezon et al., 2007] reported that in aphasic patients spontaneous recovery takes place in the first year; and for that reason, it is very important that drug therapy occurs before spontaneous recovery has taken place [de Boissezon et al., 2007].

According to de Boissezon and co-workers [2007], language improvement due to drug therapy takes place in two different ways, i.e. in a direct and indirect way. On the one hand, drug therapy improves language in a direct way if there is a significant improvement in language performance immediately after the administration of the active drug and if the achieved improvements vanish after drug withdrawal (see for instance the effects of vasopressive agents in the very acute stroke phase). On the other hand, drug therapy improves language in an indirect way, if other factors, such as spontaneous brain plasticity or effects of training, are involved in functional recovery. The achieved improvements do not vanish, even if drug therapy is interrupted (see for instance the effects of dexamphetamine). In this case, it can be hypothesized that drug therapy promotes post-stroke rec

:uronal activity in those neuronal circuits which are functionally-damaged
le Boissezon et al., 2007].

We are of the opinion that drugs interact only with particular language
functions, such as fluency and prosody which are modulated by particular
subcortical anatomical structures and neuronal pathways. We think that it is
pretty difficult that drugs are able to interact with complex language functions,
such as pragmatics and semantics, as these language functions are modulated
by various complex neuronal pathways. As mentioned previously, the
elaboration of language happens in a more distributed way in the two
hemispheres. In fact, almost the entire neocortex of the left hemisphere and in
part of the right hemisphere is involved in the elaboration of language,
including the temporal, parietal, prefrontal, and frontal lobes. Therefore, many
different neuronal networks and neurotransmitters are involved in the
elaboration of speech and language, and it is quite difficult that a particular
pharmacological agent may be able to modulate all these different
neurotransmitters and neuronal networks. The pathological processes which
affect the CNS and cause language deficits are as complex as the processes
which underlie the elaboration of speech and language. Moreover, these
pathological processes influence as many neurotransmitters and neuronal
pathways as non-pathological processes do. For that reason, it is unrealistic to
believe that a single pharmacological agent could promote language recovery.
We have noticed that significant improvements have been achieved when drug
therapy was combined with speech therapy. According to us, speech therapy is
the most important and successful tool used to improve language functions in
aphasic patients.

We think that a single-case study is the *conditio sine qua non* to
understand the effects of a particular drug on language as in this case there is a
rather simple interaction between pharmacological therapy and language
function. We investigated the effects of topiramate in a patient with a light
form of non-fluent dysphasia and partial epileptic seizures which are most
likely the after-effect of a previous craniocerebral injury. Our patient was
treated with 100mg of topiramate twice a day for three months in order to
stabilize his mood. The neuropsychological test battery was administered
during treatment with topiramate and 10 months after withdrawal of
topiramate. Moreover, our patient underwent SPECT investigation during
treatment with topiramate and 10 months after withdrawal of topiramate. We
noticed that the treatment with topiramate aggravated the pre-existent speech
and language disorder. His oral output was characterized by very long pauses
and by a severe dysprosody which compromised the normal speech fluency.

overy. But according to Martinsson and co-workers [2004], a
should not be used in clinical practice as the mortality rate is higl
treated with amphetamines than in those treated with the placebo.
According to de Boissezon and colleagues [2007], drugs wl
for treating aphasic patients should be language specific. A v
study should also include non-language measurements which ai
observe those effects which are language specific, but in this case
effects of the drug should be observed on non-language measurer
now, only very few research groups [Gupta et al., 1995; Orgo
Raymer et al., 2001; Walker-Batson et al., 2001; Tanaka et al., 2
de Boissezon et al., 2007] included non-language measurements in
but, surprisingly, they have not found any language specific effec
now, the various neuroscientific research groups could
pharmacological agents which interact with the neuronal structures
language processing [de Boissezon et al., 2007]. In addition, it is be
those neuronal structures which are involved in language processing
from particular neuronal structures which had evolved earlie
phylogenetic point of view. Therefore, it seems rather plausible
structures could share the same neuro-chemical features [de Boisse
2007]. So, according to de Boissezon and co-workers [2
pharmacological agents used for treating aphasic patients are not
specific, and the effects observed in the various studies are caus
global action of drugs on several neuronal networks which interfere
language processes. The above-mentioned viewpoint coincides with
models which tried to explain the mechanisms of drug effects. Acc
these models, the stimulation of neuronal pathways which have their
the brain stem nuclei and which ascend to various cortical areas wot
cortical activity easier, including those processes which are inv
language output [de Boissezon et al., 2007]. These models were
proposed for the dopaminergic pathways, but the various research
which applied these models to aphasia recovery did not obtain sig
results. It has to be pointed out, that the research groups which r
relevant results in group studies reported improvement of global
scores [de Boissezon et al., 2007]. Furthermore, pharmacological agents
necessarily modulate language in general; in fact, there are some clinica
in which drugs modulate only some particular language functions, s
speech fluency [Sechi, 2006; de Boissezon et al., 2007]. It seems beli
that some aphasic symptoms, such as speech fluency could be improv
pharmacological agents. In other words, it is possible that drugs impro

His language functions improved significantly after drug wash-out. The neuropsychological findings were confirmed by the SPECT investigation, i.e. there was a severe reduction of cortical tracer uptake in the left brain hemisphere and focal areas of low uptake in the right temporal and parietal lobes during therapy. The depressant effect of topiramate on tracer uptake might be related both to a primary biochemical effect by topiramate on the cortical neuronal/glial cells already lightly damaged after the previous traumatic brain injury, mainly in the left hemisphere, as documented by the MRI study, and to a diaschisis effect on remote cortical areas [Sechi et al., 1995], due to a possible depressant action of topiramate on the corticocallosal connections. But after drug wash-out, 99mTc HM-PAO uptake globally improved, particularly in the right temporal and parietal lobes and in the left fronto-parietal and temporo-parietal cortical areas. Our findings coincide with those made by other research groups [Meador et al., 2003; Gross-Tsur et al., 2004; Gomer et al., 2007]. In fact, various clinical studies [Meador et al., 2003; Gross-Tsur et al., 2004; Gomer et al., 2007] demonstrated that topiramate has a variety of cognitive side effects which range from psychomotor slowing, memory and attentional problems to slow information processing and poor performance in verbal fluency tasks. Furthermore, our findings provide evidence that pharmacological agents interact only with some particular language functions and not with language in general. The language system and the neuronal pathways which are involved in the elaboration of language are far too complex to be modulated by a pharmacological agent.

In order to obtain the best possible results, it is very important that patients who are included in a study are screened carefully, i.e. various factors, such as lesions (location, size, aetiology, and time post-stroke), patients (age, gender, handedness, education level, and mood disorder), aphasia (severity, typology, and spontaneous recover), and speech therapy (type, exercise difficulty, duration, and patient personal implication) can determine the success of a pharmacological therapy [de Boissezon et al., 2007].

In conclusion, it has to be pointed out that further well-designed, randomized, double-blind, placebo-controlled clinical trials which are carried out in combination with speech therapy are needed not only to understand the mechanisms which underlie language recovery but also to find an adequate therapy for aphasic patients.

REFERENCES

Ackermann, H. (2008). Cerebellar contributions to speech production and speech perception: psycholinguistic and neurobiological perspectives. *Trends in Neuroscience, 31*(6), 265-272.

Albert, M. L., Bachman, D. L., Morgan, A. & Helm-Estabrooks, N. (1988). Pharmacotherapy for aphasia. *Neurology, 38*, 877-789.

Albert, M. L., Goodglass, H., Helm, N. A., Rubens, A. B. & Alexander, M. P. (1972). *Clinical aspects of dysphasia.* Vienna, Springer Verlag.

Alexander, G. A. (1994). Basal ganglia-thalamocortical circuits: Their role in control of movement. *J. Clin. Neurophysiol, 11*, 420-431.

Amaducci, L., Sorbi, S., Albanese, A. & Gainotti, G. (1981). Choline acetyltransferase (ChAT) activity differs in right and left human temporal lobes. *Neurology, 31*, 799-805.

Amunts, K., Weiss, P. H., Mohlberg, H., Pieperhoff, P., Eickhoff, S., Gurd, J. M., Marshall, J. C., Shah, N. J., Fink, G. R. & Zilles, K. (2004). Analysis of neural mechanisms underlying verbal fluency in cytoarchitectonically defined stereotaxic space – The roles of Brodmann areas 44 and 45. *NeuroImage, 22*, 42-56.

Ashtary, F., Janghorbani, M., Chitsaz, A., Reisi, M. & Bahrami, A. (2006). A randomized, double-blind trial of bromocriptine efficacy in non-fluent aphasia after stroke. *Neurology, 66*, 914-916.

Barrett, A. M. & Eslinger, P. J. (2007). Amantadine for Adynamic Speech. Possible Benefit for Aphasia? *Am. J. Phs. Med. Rehabil, 68*, 605-612.

Basso, A. (2005). *Conoscere e rieducare l'afasia.* Roma, Il Pensiero Scientifico Editore.

Berthier, M. L., Green, C., Higueras, C., Fernández, I., Hinojosa, J. & Martín, M. C. (2006). A randomized, placebo-controlled study of donepezil in poststroke aphasia. *Neurology, 67,* 1687-1689.

Bhatia, K. P. & Marsden, D. (1994). The behavioural and motor consequences of focal lesions of the basal ganglia in man. *Brain, 117,* 859-876.

Bragoni, M., Altieri, M., Di Pietro, V., Padovani, A., Mostardini, C. & Lenzi, G. L. (2000). Bromocriptine and speech therapy in non-fluent chronic aphasia after stroke. *Neurol. Sci, 21,* 19-22.

Brody, T. M., Larner, J., Minneman, K. P. & Neu, H. C. (1994). *Human Pharmacology. Molecular to Clinical.* St. Louis – Missouri, Mosby-Year Book, Inc.

Brunner, R. J., Kornhuber, H. H., Seemüller, E., Suger, G. & Wallesch, C. W. (1982). Basal ganglia participation in language pathology. *Brain Lang, 16,* 281-299.

Cacciari, C. (2001). *Psicologia del Linguaggio.* Bologna, Il Mulino.

Caplan, D. (1998). *Neurolinguistics and linguistic aphasiology. An introduction.* Cambridge, Cambridge University Press.

Cappa, S. F. (1997). Subcortical aphasia: still a useful concept? *Brain Lang, 58,* 424-426.

Catani, M., Jones, D. K. & H. ffytche, D. (2005). Perisylvian language networks of the human brain. *Ann. Neurol, 57,* 8-16.

Christensen, T. A., Antonucci, S. M., Lockwood, J. L., Kittleson, M. & Plante, E. (2008). Cortical and subcortical contributions to the attentive processing of speech. *NeuroReport, 19,* 1101-1105.

Ciurli, P., Marangolo, P. & Basso, A. (1996). *Esame del Linguaggio-II.* Firenze, Organizzazioni Speciali.

Cooper, J. R., Bloom, F. E. & Roth, R. H. (2003). *The Biochemical Basis of Neuropharmacology.* New York, Oxford University Press.

Copland, D. (2001). Discourse priming of homophones in individuals with dominant nonthalamic subcortical lesions, cortical lesions and Parkinson's disease. *J. Clin. Exp. Neuropsychol, 23,* 538-556.

Copland, D. (2003). The basal ganglia and semantic engagement. Potential insights from semantic priming in individuals with subcortical vascular lesions, Parkinson's disease and cortical lesions. *J. Int. Neuropsychol. Soc, 9,* 1041-1052

Crosson, B. (1997). Models of subcortical functions in language: current status. *J. Neurolinguist, 10,* 277-300.

Crosson, B. (2002). Basal Ganglia. In: V. S. Ramachandran (Ed.), *Encyclopedia of the Human Brain*, vol. 1-4 (pp. 367-379). San Diego, Academic Press.

Cummings, J. L, Darkins, A., Mendez, M., Hill, M. A. & Benson, D. F. (1988). Alzheimer's disease and Parkinson's disease: comparison of speech and language alterations. *Neurology, 38*, 680-684.

Damasio, A. R., Damasio, H., Rizzo, M., Varney, N. & Gersh, F. (1982). Aphasia with non-hemorrhagic lesions in the basal ganglia and internal capsule. *Arch. Neurol, 39*, 15-24.

de Boissezon, X., Peran, P. de Boysson, C. & Démonet, J. F. (2007). Pharmacotherapy of aphasia: Myth or reality? *Brain and Language, 102*, 114-125.

Démonet, J. F., Thierry, G. & Cardebat, D. (2005). Renewal of the neurophysiology of language: Functional neuroimaging. *Physiol. Rev, 85*, 49-95.

Fabbro, F. (1999). *The neurolinguistics of bilingualism. An introduction.* Hove and New York, Psychology Press.

Ferstl, E. C., Neumann, J., Bogler, C. & von Cramon, D. Y. (2008). The extended language network: a meta-analysis of neuroimaging studies on text comprehension. *Human Brain Mapping, 234*, 53-63.

Glick, S., Ross, D. & Hough, L. (1982). Lateral asymmetry of neurotransmitters in human brain. *Brain Res, 6*, 260-270.

Gordon, W. P. & Illes, J. (1987). Neurolinguistic characteristics of language production in Huntington's disease: a preliminary report. *Brain Lang, 31*, 1-10.

Gomer, B., Wagner, K., Frings, L., Saar, J., Carius, A., Härle, M., Steinhoff, B. J. & Schulze-Bonhage, A. (2007). The influence of antiepileptic drugs on cognition: A comparison of levetiracetam with topiramate. *Epilepsy & Behavior, 10*, 486-494.

Grossman, M. (1999). Sentence processing in Parkinson's disease. *Brain Cogn, 40*, 387-413.

Gross-Tsur, V. & Shalev, R. (2004). Reversible language regression as an adverse effect of topiramate treatment in children. *Neurology, 62*, 299-300.

Gupta, S. R., Mlcoch, A. G., Scolaro, C. & Moritz, T. (1995). Bromocriptine treatment of non-fluent aphasia. *Neurology, 45*, 2170-2173.

Hardman, J. G., Limbird, L. E. & Goodman-Gilman, A. (2001). *Goodman & Gilman's – The Pharmacological Basis of Therapeutics.* New York, McGraw-Hill.

Huber, W. (1999). The Role of Piracetam in the Treatment of Acute and Chronic Aphasia. *Pharmacopsychiat, 32*, 38-43.

Hutsler, J. J. & Gazzaniga, M. S. (1996). Acetylcholinesterase staining in human auditory and language cortices: regional variation of structural features. *Cereb Cortex, 6*, 260-270.

Illes, J. (1989). Neurolinguistic features of spontaneous language production dissociate three forms of neurodegenerative disease: Alzheimer's, Huntington's, and Parkinson's. *Brain Lang, 37*, 628-642.

Kandel, E. R., Schwartz, J. H. & Jessell, T. M. (2000). *Principles of neural sciences* (4th Edition). New York, McGraw-Hill.

Katzung, B. G. (2007). *Basic and Clinical Pharmacology*. New York, McGraw-Hill.

Ketteler, D., Kastrau, F., Vohn, R. & Huber, W. (2008). The subcortical role of language processing. High level linguistic features such as ambiguity-resolution and the human brain; an fMRI study. *NeuroImage, 39*, 2002-2009.

Klein, R. B. & Albert, M. L. (2004). Can Drug Therapies Improve Language Functions of Individuals with Aphasia? A Review of the Evidence. *Seminars in Speech and Language, 25*, 193-204.

Làdavas, E. & Berti, A. (2002). *Neuropsicologia*. Bologna, Il Mulino.

Lieberman, P., Friedman, J. & Feldman, L. S. (1990). Syntax comprehension deficits in Parkinson's disease. *J. Nerv. Ment. Dis, 178*, 360-365.

Long, D. & Young, J. (2003). Dexamphetamine treatment in stroke. *Q. J. Med, 96*, 673-685.

Martinsson, L. & Eksborg, S. (2004). Drugs for Stroke Recovery. The Example of Amphetamines. *Drugs Aging, 21*, 67-79.

McNamara, P., Krueger, M., O'Quin, K., Clark, J. & Durso, R. (1996). Grammaticality judgments and sentence comprehension in Parkinson's disease: a comparison with Broca's aphasia. *Int. J. Neurosci, 86*, 151-166.

McNamara, P. & Durso, R. (2000). Language functions in Parkinson's disease: evidence for a neurochemistry of language. In: L. T. Connor, & L. K. Obler, L.K. (Eds.), *Neurobehaviour of Language and Cognition. Studies of Normal Aging and Brain Damage* (pp. 201-212). Boston, MA, Wolters.

McNamara, P. & Albert, M. L. (2004). Neuropharmacology of Verbal Perseveration. *Seminars in Speech and Language, 25*, 309-320.

Meador, K. J., Loring, D. W., Hulihan, J. F., Kamin, M. & Karim, R. (2003). Differential cognitive and behavioural effects of topiramate and valproate. *Neurology, 60*, 1483-1488.

Nadeau, S. E. & Crosson, B. (1997). Subcortical aphasia. *Brain Lang.*, *58*, 355-402.

Nadeau, S. E., Gonzalez-Rothi, L. J. & Crosson, B. (2000). *Aphasia and Language. Theory to Practice.* New York, Guilford Press.

Naeser, M. A., Alexander, M. P., Helm-Estabrooks, N., Levine, H. L., Laughlin, S. A. & Geschwind, N. (1982). Aphasia with predominantly subcortical lesion sites: description of three capsular/putaminal aphasia syndromes. *Arch. Neurol*, *39*, 2-14.

Natsopoulos D., Katsarou, Z., Bostantzopoulou, S., Grouios, G., Mentenopoulos, G. & Logothetis, J. (1991). Strategies in comprehension of relative clauses by parkinsonian patients. *Cortex*, *27*, 255-268.

Natsopoulos D., Grouios, G., Bostantzopoulou, S., Mentenopoulos, G., Katsarou, Z. & Logothetis, J. (1993). Algorithmic and heuristic strategies in comprehension of complement clauses by patients with Parkinson's disease. *Neuropsychologia*, *31*, 951-964.

Paradis, M. (2004). *A neurolinguistic theory of bilingualism.* Amsterdam, John Benjamins.

Piazzini, A., Chifari, R., Canevini, M. P., Turner, K., Fontana, S. P. & Canger, R. (2006). Levetiracetam: An improvement of attention and of oral fluency in patients with partial epilepsy. *Epilepsy Research*, *68*, 181-188.

Pinker, S. & Ullman, M. T. (2002). The past and future of the past tense. *Trends Cogn. Sci*, *6*, 456-463.

Poeppel, D. & Hickok, G. (2004).Towards a new functional anatomy of language. *Cognition*, *92*, 1-12.

Schatzberg, A. F. & Nemeroff, C. B. (2001). *Essentials of Clinical Psychopharmacology.* Washington, D.C., American Psychiatric Publishing, Inc.

Sechi, G. P., Casu, A. R., Rosati, G., Spanu, A., Deserra, F., Nuvoli, S., Deiana, G. A. & Madeddu, G. (1995). Cerebral and cerebellar diaschisis following carbamazepine therapy. *Prog. Neuro-Psychopharmacol. & Biol. Psychiat*, *19*, 889-901.

Sechi, G. P., Cocco, G. A., D'Onofrio, M., Deriu, M. G. & Rosati, G. (2006). Disfluent speech in patients with partial epilepsy: Beneficial effect of levetiracetam. *Epilepsy & Behavior*, *9*, 521-523.

Siegel, G. J., Albers, R. W., Brady, S. T. & Price, D. L. (2006). *Basic Neurochemistry. Molecular, Cellular, and Medical Aspects.* London, Academic Press.

Small, S. (1994). Pharmacotherapy of Aphasia. A Critical Review. *Stroke*, *25*, 1282-1289.

Sommer, I. E., Oranje, B., Ramsey, N. F., Klerk, F. A., Mandl, R. C. W., Westenberg, H. G. M. & Kahn, R. (2005). The influence of amphetamine on language activation: an fMRI study. *Psychopharmacology*, *183*, 387-393.

Ullman, M. T. (2001). A neurocognitive perspective on language: the Declarative/ Procedural Model. *Nat. Rev. Neurosci*, *2*, 717-726.

Ullman, M. T., Corkin, S., Coppola, M., Hickok, G., Growdon, J. H. & Koroshetz, W. J. (1997). A neural dissociation within language: evidence that the mental dictionary is part of declarative memory, and that grammatical rules are processed by the procedural system. *J. Cogn. Neurosci*, *9*, 266-276.

Vigneau, M., Beaucousin, V., Hervé, P. Y., Duffau, H., Crivello, F., Houdé, O., Mazoyer, B. & Tzourio-Mazoyer, N. (2006). Meta-analyzing left hemisphere language areas: Phonology, semantics, and sentence processing. *NeuroImage*, *30*, 1414-1432.

Wallesch, C. W., Kornhuber, H. H., Brunner, R. J., Kunz, T., Hollerbach, B. & Suger, G. (1983). Lesions of the basal ganglia, thalamus, and deep white matter: differential effects on language functions. *Brain Lang*, *20*, 286-304.

Wallesch, C. W. & Papagno, C. (1988). Subcortical aphasia. In F. Clifford Rose, R. Whurr, & M. A. Wyke (Eds.), *Aphasia* (pp. 257-287). London, Whurr.

Wallesch, C. W. (1997). Symptomatology of subcortical aphasia. *J. Neurolinguist*, *10*, 267-275.

Wernicke, C. (1874). *Der Aphasische Symptomencomplex. Eine Psychologische Studie auf anatomischer Basis*. Breslau, Max Cohn & Weigert.

Whiting, E., Chenery, H. J., Chalk, J. & Copland, D. (2007). Dexamphetamine boosts naming treatment effects in chronic aphasia. *JINS*, *13*, 972-979.

Zanetti, D. (2009). Bilingual aphasia. Adaptation of the Bilingual Aphasia Test (BAT) to Sardinian and study of a clinical case. *Unpublished Ph.D. Thesis* – Università degli Studi di Sassari.

INDEX

M

N

O

P

V

T

W